Genetic Influences on Response to Drug Treatment for Major Psychiatric Disorders

Janusz K. Rybakowski • Alessandro Serretti

Editors

Genetic Influences on Response to Drug Treatment for Major Psychiatric Disorders

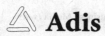 **Adis**

Editors
Janusz K. Rybakowski
Department of Adult Psychiatry
Poznan University of Medical Sciences
Poznan
Poland

Alessandro Serretti
Department of Biomedical and Neuromotor
Sciences
University of Bologna
Bologna
Italy

ISBN 978-3-319-27038-8   ISBN 978-3-319-27040-1   (eBook)
DOI 10.1007/978-3-319-27040-1

Library of Congress Control Number: 2016930560

Springer Cham Heidelberg New York Dordrecht London

Printed on acid-free paper

Adis is a brand of Springer
Springer International Publishing AG Switzerland is part of Springer Science+Business Media (www.springer.com)

Introduction

Psychiatric disorders affect a significant percentage of the population, making the issue of their optimal treatment an extremely important one. A judicious use of pharmacological treatment would be the most appropriate and effective method of help to most of such patients. Interindividual genetic variations can influence the responses of patients to any psychotropic medications; therefore, the results of studies investigating genetic background of such a mechanism could facilitate the effectiveness of the treatment.

Pharmacogenetics of the treatment of psychiatric disorders has become a rapidly expanding area in the last two decades. This has been mostly caused by the introduction of molecular genetic methods to the field. The most used approach for pharmacogenetic studies of efficacy and safety of treatment with individual drugs is still a "candidate gene" method. However, recently, genome-wide association studies (GWAS) have also been entering into this subject, exemplified in this book by the GWAS of lithium response in bipolar disorder. Due to the progress in molecular genetics employed for estimating psychotropic drug response, "pharmacogenetics", which assesses genetically determined interindividual differences in response to drugs, has been gradually becoming "pharmacogenomics", which uses genome-based technologies for this purpose.

The issue of pharmacogenetics (pharmacogenomics) of psychiatric disorders has been recently covered by several books, the most important ones published in 2010–2011. The first book to mention is *Psychiatric Pharmacogenomics*, published in 2010 and authored by the late David Mrazek (1948–2013). The idea of the book is an original one, showing a contribution of 14 genes (four cytochrome genes, three neurotransmitter transporter genes, three serotonin receptor genes, and three dopamine receptor genes) to response of psychotropic drugs in various psychiatric diseases. Another book, published in 2010, came within the Karger series of *Advances in Biological Psychiatry*, titled *Pharmacogenomics in Psychiatry*, and edited by Matthias Schwab, Wolfgang Kaschka, and Eduardo Spina. In this book, the pharmacogenomic findings in individual psychiatric conditions, such as schizophrenia, depression, attention-deficit/hyperactivity disorder, eating disorders, and personality disorders, have been reviewed. And finally, in 2011, the last edition of

Bernard Lerer's book, *Pharmacogenetics of Psychotropic Drugs*, which was first published in 2002, was released. This is the most comprehensive publication, covering both the clinical and molecular background of this topic, as well as pharmacogenetics of specific psychotropic drugs and disorders.

Several years have passed since the publication of these books, and the aim of this one is to cover the major developments in pharmacogenetics and pharmacogenomics of major psychoses in the last two decades, including also the period 2010–2015. However, the book we are presenting here is unique in several aspects compared with the books mentioned previously. Written by global experts, this book provides a modern comprehensive insight into the pharmacogenetics of treatment of major psychoses: schizophrenia, bipolar disorder, and depression. Secondly, the pharmacogenomics of three categories of the most important psychiatric drugs such as antipsychotics, antidepressants, and mood stabilizers has been updated and reviewed. From the point of view of mainstream psychiatry, both these diagnostic and drug categories have made the most significant topics in recent years.

The main practical aim of pharmacogenetics and pharmacogenomics of psychotropic drugs is to make drug treatments in psychiatric medicine more effective in individual patients. Therefore, a related issue to pharmacogenetics in psychiatry is that of personalized medicine. This model proposes that each medical intervention (e.g., pharmacotherapy) should be tailored to the individual patient. The term personalized medicine was first coined in the context of genetics; thus, the use of genetic information about pharmacotherapy (i.e., pharmacogenetics) makes the most important contribution to this field. Although this model has still not been widely used in psychiatry, the amount of pharmacogenetic data presented in this book may greatly contribute to reaching clinical practice by personalized prescription in the not so distant future. There is a significant role of modern psychiatric pharmacogenetics to meet such expectations.

Apart from providing a timely overview of what has been achieved in the area of psychiatric pharmacogenomics in the last two decades, this book also mentions some promising directions and perspectives for future research. The first direction is connected with the development of molecular genetics. The GWAS study of lithium response in bipolar disorder has been already performed, and such research with other drugs used in major psychoses could be possible in the future. Other developments in this field such as microarray technologies and sequencing techniques may be shortly available for the pharmacogenomics of psychotropic drugs. Also, the studies of epigenetic mechanisms such as DNA methylation, histone modification, and regulation by miRNA have been gradually introduced in pharmacogenetic research. Another area of research is linking pharmacogenetic assessment with biomarkers, including neuroimaging ones. Studies exemplifying such approach in depression were reviewed in a chapter of this book.

Finally, the attempts to use pharmacogenetics of antipsychotic, antidepressant, and mood-stabilizing drugs in practice are presented in the last chapter of the book. The clinical utility of pharmacogenomic testing has been evolving; although, at a slower pace than it has been anticipated. We are just on the threshold of introducing new pharmacogenetic tools for psychiatric practice, and one of such test (GeneSight) is now reimbursed by Medicare in the USA. It may be expected that several other tools of this kind will enter psychiatric practice in the next years.

We sincerely hope that reading this book, many physicians (mostly psychiatrists) and pharmacologists, as well as all those engaged in clinical and experimental neuroscience, will find it useful; not only as an update to present art of knowledge in pharmacogenetics of drugs used in major psychoses but also for providing new insights into the development and applications of pharmacogenomics in psychiatry.

Poznan, Poland   Janusz K. Rybakowski
Bologna, Italy   Alessandro Serretti

Contents

Chapter 1
Pharmacogenetics of the Efficacy of Antipsychotic Drugs in Schizophrenia

María J. Arranz, Josefina Perez Blanco, and Barbara Arias Samperiz

Abstract Response to pharmacotherapy is highly variable, complex and difficult to predict. Genetic factors influence, at least partially, clinical response to drugs. It has been proposed that the use of genetic information may help to predict patient's response to medications. In the last decades, pharmacogenetic studies have produced numerous reports of genetic associations with treatment efficacy and related side effects. However, only a limited number of these findings may have clinical utility in psychiatry. In this chapter, we will review pharmacogenetic findings in relation to common antipsychotic drugs used for the treatment of schizophrenia and discuss their clinical applicability.

1.1 Introduction

1.1.1 Pharmacogenetics of Antipsychotic Efficacy

Antipsychotic drugs are the mainstay treatment for severe psychotic episodes of schizophrenia. However, the large proportion of failures and the severity of induced side effects reinforce the need for personalised treatment. Genetic information has been proposed as a tool to help in the management of antipsychotic treatment. New genotyping technologies, cheaper and faster, have facilitated the identification of a number of genes involved in pharmacokinetic and pharmacodynamic processes that

M.J. Arranz, PhD (✉)
Fundació Docència i Recerca Mútua Terrassa, c/Sant Antoni, 19, Terrassa 08221, Spain

Department of Psychiatry – CIBERSAM, Hospital de la Santa Creu i Sant Pau,
Barcelona, Spain
e-mail: mjarranz@mutuaterrassa.es; maria.arranz@kcl.ac.uk

J.P. Blanco, MD
Department of Psychiatry – CIBERSAM, Hospital de la Santa Creu i Sant Pau,
Barcelona, Spain

B.A. Samperiz
Department of Anthropology, University of Barcelona, Barcelona, Spain

© Springer International Publishing Switzerland 2016
J.K. Rybakowski, A. Serretti (eds.), *Genetic Influences on Response to Drug Treatment for Major Psychiatric Disorders*, DOI 10.1007/978-3-319-27040-1_1

1

contribute to the variability observed in response to pharmacotherapy. Decades of pharmacogenetic research on antipsychotics have produced interesting results, although few findings have a clear clinical value. In addition, pharmacogenetic research has contributed information on the mechanisms of action of currently available antipsychotic drugs. However, the application of pharmacogenetic knowledge to improve antipsychotic efficacy and safety or in the development of new drugs is limited. This chapter summarises the genetic findings in relation to antipsychotic efficacy and induced side effects, the clinical applications of these findings and the current steps taken to introduce their use in clinical settings.

1.1.2 Clinical Response Phenotypes

Undoubtedly, one of the main challenges in the field is the difficulty in determining clinical response to antipsychotic treatment. The assessment of clinical outcome is complex. Aside from genetic factors, clinical, demographic and environmental factors influence treatment outcome. Factors relevant to drug treatment, including antipsychotic type, treatment adherence and duration, and concomitant medications, contribute to response variability [14]. Clinical factors such as baseline severity, duration of untreated psychosis, comorbidities and age of onset are directly related to treatment efficacy. Environmental factors such us diet, smoking habits and concomitant treatments amongst others play a role on drug availability [9, 14]. Finally, the age and ethnic group of the patient may also contribute to treatment variability and should be taken into account when conducting genetic association studies. In addition, response criterion is not universally standardised. Whereas a threshold of 20–30 % improvement in PANSS scores is a widely used criteria, other response definitions such as improvement in global assessment scores (GAS) are considered. All these factors and criteria variability complicate the reliability and reproducibility of pharmacogenetic studies.

1.1.3 Research Strategies

Research to identify treatment-related genetic factors has relied mainly on candidate genes association studies. In these studies, the allelic and genotypic frequencies of candidate gene variants are compared between patients responding to treatment and non-responding patients, or tested versus the level of improvement observed in treated patient. This strategy has achieved the identification of a number of response biomarkers with clinical applicability which are described in the following sections. However, candidate gene approaches have had little impact on discerning the mechanism of action of antipsychotic drugs as candidate genes are selected from previous knowledge. So far, candidate gene studies have identified genetic variants in known drug targets and in CYP metabolic enzymes as important factors influencing response variability [38, 83]. Thus, rather than providing new information, these studies have confirmed previous knowledge, which could be used for the identification of patients likely to respond to treatment and/or likely to develop side effects.

The development of high-throughput genotyping techniques facilitated the introduction of genomic strategies into psychiatric research. These strategies do not require previous knowledge or specific hypothesis as the entire genome, epigenome or transcriptome is interrogated by genome-wide (GWAS), epigenome-wide (EWAS) and transcriptomic association studies, respectively. These studies have the capability to produce novel information on the antipsychotics' mechanism of action that could be used to develop improved treatments. However, these strategies have had a moderate success in psychiatry. The difficulty of obtaining large cohorts of schizophrenia patients on antipsychotic monotherapy with accurate measurements of clinical change during treatment is the main obstacle encountered. Although several novel associations have been observed using these strategies (see Sect. 1.2.2), their reliability needs to be confirmed in independent studies before the information can be used clinically.

1.2 Pharmacogenetic and Pharmacogenomic Findings

1.2.1 Candidate Gene Studies

Numerous response-related genes have been discovered using a candidate gene approach. However, findings have rarely been universally replicated. Differences in the treatment duration, sample size, assessment method, population group and antipsychotic type may partially explain discrepancies between studies [11]. Nevertheless, several findings have been confirmed in independent studies and can be considered true findings. Table 1.2 summarises findings related to drug targets and side effects. In many occasions, drug-target genes and their variants are reportedly associated with both the level of treatment efficacy and with drug adverse reactions, although there are several genes that have been only associated to antipsychotic-induced adverse reactions. This is a clear indication that current antipsychotic treatment could be improved by developing new drugs with specific targets of proved therapeutic value. The following sections describe the information provided by pharmacogenetic research in relation to pharmacodynamic targets and metabolic pathways and their genetic association with treatment variability.

1.2.1.1 Findings Related to Antipsychotic Efficacy

After the successful introduction of chlorpromazine as an antipsychotic in the 1950s, different antipsychotic types have been developed in an attempt to improve treatment outcome. However, the precise mechanism of action of currently

Table 1.1 Brief description of pharmacodynamic profile and main metabolic pathways of commonly used antipsychotic drugs

	Pharmacodynamic profile	Pharmacokinetic profile
Haloperidol	D2, D3, D4	CYP2D6, CYP3A4
Chlorpromazine	D2, D3, D4, 5-HT2A, 5-HT2C, 5-HT6	CYP2D6, CYP1A2
Clozapine	5-HT2A, 5-HT2C, 5-HT6, D4, D2, H1, M1, ADR1A	CYP1A2, CYP3A4, CYPD2D6, CYP2C19
Olanzapine	5-HT2A, 5-HT2C, 5-HT6, D2, D3, D4, H1, M1, ADR1A	CYP1A2, CYP2D6
Risperidone	5-HT2A, 5-HT2C, D2, D3, D4, ADR1A	CYP2D6, CYP3A4

available antipsychotic drugs remains unclear. Genetic factors can affect both the pharmacodynamic and pharmacokinetic properties of antipsychotics. Genetic alterations may cause under-expression or malfunctioning of targeted receptors and neurotransmitters. Similarly, genetic variants may alter the metabolic rates of enzymes responsible for the drugs' pharmacokinetics. Whereas antipsychotics' pharmacodynamics and pharmacokinetic properties are specifically described elsewhere, Table 1.1 briefly summarises the pharmacodynamic and pharmacokinetic profiles of commonly used antipsychotic medications.

Findings in Targeted Neurotransmitters and Transporters

First-generation antipsychotics (FGAs), resembling haloperidol and chlorpromazine, display high affinity for dopamine receptors, whereas second-generation antipsychotics (SGA) display preferential affinity for dopamine and serotonin receptors, amongst others. Numerous studies have investigated genetic variants in targeted neurotransmitters and transporters with varying results (see Table 1.2). It is important to note that Table 1.2 summarises only significant findings and that the many non-significant reports published to date are not included. However, given the difficulty of obtaining clinical samples for pharmacogenetic studies, and the complexity of response definition, when an association report is replicated in independent clinical settings, it may constitute a true finding.

The most replicated findings indicate that dopamine and serotonin genetic variants are involved in both the level of efficacy and the risk of adverse reactions. In particular, genetic variants in dopamine type 2 (D2), dopamine type 3 (D3) and serotonin type 2A (5-HT2A) are the most frequently associated with treatment efficacy [8, 14]. Dopaminergic variants are associated with response to FGA and SGA, whereas serotonergic variants are more likely to be associated with the level of efficacy of SGA, reflecting perhaps their pharmacological profiles. In general, those genetic variants associated with lower receptor expression (e.g. D2 -141-*Del*) or altered functioning (e.g. 5-HT2A 452Tyr) are associated with poorer antipsychotic efficacy [12, 14], indicating that the harbouring receptors are implicated, at least

Table 1.2 Summary of significant pharmacogenetic findings on antipsychotic medications

Gene	Associations with efficacy	Associations with side effects
Drug-targeted receptors		
ADRA1A		TD, weight gain
ADRA2A		Weight gain
D1	Clozapine, others	
D2	Clozapine, risperidone, aripiprazole, haloperidol, chlorpromazine	TD, rigidity, akathisia, weight gain, Parkinsonism, sexual dysfunction
D3	Clozapine, olanzapine, risperidone	TD, EPS, AIMS scores
D4	Clozapine, FGA	TD, weight gain
H2	Clozapine	
H3	Risperidone	
H4	Risperidone	
5-HT1A	Risperidone, SGA	
5-HT2A	Clozapine, risperidone, FGA, SGA, olanzapine	TD, weight gain, obesity
5-HT2C	Clozapine	TD, weight gain, Parkinsonism, metabolic syndrome
5-HT6	Clozapine, risperidone	Weight gain
5-HT3A	Risperidone, clozapine	
Neurotransmitter transporters		
DAT	Clozapine, others	TD, EPS
5-HTT	Clozapine, olanzapine, risperidone	Weight gain, obesity
Hepatic enzymes		
CYP1A2	Clozapine	TD, seizures, adverse reactions
CYP2D6	SGA	TD, weight gain
CYP2C9		Somnolence
CYP3A4	Risperidone	
Others		
ADRB2		EPS
COMT	Clozapine, olanzapine, risperidone	TD, Parkinsonism
BDNF	Risperidone, others	TD, weight gain
GRM3	Olanzapine, risperidone	
MDR1	Olanzapine, risperidone, bromperidol, clozapine, quetiapine	Movement disorders, weight gain
MTHFR	SGA	Metabolic syndrome
RGS2		Parkinsonism, EPS
RGS4	Risperidone	
LEP		Weight gain, dyslipidemia
LEPR		Obesity, dyslipidemia
MC4R		Weight gain
CNR1		Weight gain, metabolic syndrome, TD

Abbreviations: *TD* tardive dyskinesia, *EPS* extrapyramidal symptoms, *FGA* first-generation antipsychotics, *SGA* second-generation antipsychotics partially, in the antipsychotic mechanism of action. Genetic variants in dopamine receptors type 1 (D1) and 4 (D4) and in serotonin receptors type 1, 2C, 3 and 6 (5-HT1, 5-HT2C, 5-HT3 and 5-HT6, respectively) have also been associated with treatment efficacy, although the amount of evidence is limited [13, 14, 74, 76]. Their contribution to treatment efficacy needs clarification. Existing reports of other targeted receptors such as histamine type 2 (H2), histamine type 3 (H3) and histamine type 4 (H4) [68, 87, 88] require replication in independent cohorts to confirm their validity. Several neurotransmitter transporter variants have also been linked to treatment variability. The most significant finding indicates that the serotonin transporter (5-HTT) gene harbours polymorphic variants that influence the level of efficacy of the SGA clozapine, olanzapine and risperidone [10, 17, 20, 53, 86], providing further evidence of the important role of the serotonergic system in antipsychotic activity. Interestingly, studies have also linked variants in the dopamine transporter (DAT1) gene [17], but this finding needs confirmation.

Notwithstanding the numerous studies failing to replicate these findings, taken globally, these results indicate that the dopamine and serotonin systems play a major role in the therapeutic activity of currently available antipsychotics. This information may be useful to select patients who can benefit from available medications in a personalised manner. However, pharmacogenetic studies indicate that other targeted neurotransmitter pathways such as the adrenergic, glutamatergic, histaminic and muscarinic systems do not play a major role in the mechanism of action of current drugs. These receptor systems may be valid therapeutic targets, and novel drugs targeting glutamatergic receptors and other genes directly linked to risk of schizophrenia are under investigation [44].

Findings in Metabolic Enzymes

The cytochrome P450 (CYP) group of metabolic enzymes are responsible for the biotransformation and clearance of more than 80 % of drugs, including antipsychotic medications. Table 1.1 summarises the main metabolic pathways of commonly used antipsychotics. It is well known that the genes encoding for these hepatic enzymes may harbour functional polymorphisms that render the enzymes inactive or poor metabolisers (PM), or induce higher metabolic rates (ultrarapid metabolisers, UM). These polymorphisms have consistently been associated with drug plasma concentrations [18, 23, 30, 81, 91], with individuals with one or more PM copies presenting higher plasma levels of substrate drugs than normal metabolisers (EM) and individuals with UM presenting lower plasma concentrations of drug metabolites. Alterations in genes controlling antipsychotics' clearance can have a direct impact on treatment efficacy. Low drug plasma levels caused by the presence of UMs may lead to poor response. Additionally, the presence of PMs and, in some cases, UMs has been associated with toxic reactions, leading to side effects. This, in turn, may lead to poor compliance and lack of response. Several studies have reported associations between CYP polymorphisms and variability in the response to antidepressant medications [63, 77, 83]. However, little evidence relating CYP functional variants and level of antipsychotic efficacy can be found in the literature. CYP1A2 UM variants have been associated with low plasma levels and lack of therapeutic response to clozapine [33], whereas CYP2D6 and CYP3A4 variants were associated with response to SGA [23, 32]. The singularity of these findings and the moderate sample size warrants further investigation. The availability of different metabolic pathways may serve to explain the low impact that functional metabolic polymorphisms seem to have on antipsychotic efficacy.

Others

Aside from targeted receptors and hepatic enzymes, a number of genes including metabolic enzymes, transporters and genes directly linked to schizophrenia have been associated to treatment response. The most biologically relevant findings associate polymorphisms in catechol-o-methyltransferase (COMT) and multidrug resistance 1 (MDR1) genes with antipsychotic response. COMT is an enzyme involved in the metabolic degradation of catecholamines, including dopamine catabolism, and is located in a region linked to mental disorders. The COMT gene harbours a well-investigated functional polymorphism, Val158Met. The COMT Met158 variant displays lower enzymatic activity which leads to higher dopamine availability. Interestingly, this variant is associated with higher improvement in response to SGA treatments [7, 16, 71, 89, 97], suggesting that control of dopamine activity is part of their antipsychotic action. MDR1, also known as ABCB1, is a transmembrane protein that regulates blood-brain barrier transport. Genetic variants in this transporter have been associated with the level of efficacy of several antipsychotic drugs [19, 62, 73, 92, 93] and may reflect drug availability in the brain. BDNF is another protein which has been linked to schizophrenia risk and recent studies have also been related to response levels [56, 95]. Finally, the evidence supporting the association between glutamate metabotropic receptor type 3 (GRM3), methylenetetrahydrofolate reductase (MTHFR) and regulator of G-protein signalling 4 (RGS4) genetic variants with level of efficacy is limited and needs replication [48, 58].

In summary, several genes coding for targeted receptors, transporters and enzymes have been shown to contain genetic variants that significantly influence the level of antipsychotic efficacy. However, the magnitude of these associations is moderate and therefore their clinical value limited. Single individual genes or variants cannot be used for the personalisation of antipsychotic treatment, given the low genetic effects observed. Attempts at combining information in several genes, and with clinical and environmental data, have not produced the clear results required for the application of this information into clinical practice [10, 14, 57]. Standardisation of treatment response definition and further studies including detailed clinical and environmental data are required to move the field forward before using this knowledge for the prediction of the level of efficacy of currently available antipsychotic treatments.

1.2.1.2 Findings Related to Antipsychotic-Induced Side Effects

Whereas research protocols for the measurement of clinical efficacy are still in need of standardisation, side effects constitute less complex phenotypes which are relatively easier to determine (e.g. amount of weight gain, presence/absence of movement disorders). Given the severity of the side effects associated with antipsychotic treatment, it is not surprising that in recent years relatively more effort has been put into identifying side-effect biomarkers. As a result, pharmacogenetic studies have been relatively more successful in finding genetic factors contributing to adverse reactions than in finding response-related variants. As in the case of level of efficacy, genes involved in pharmacodynamics and pharmacokinetic processes, and genes previously linked with schizophrenia risk, have been related to a variety of antipsychotic-induced side effects. The most significant findings are summarised in the following subsections.

Findings in Targeted Neurotransmitter Receptors and Transporters

As in the case of treatment response, pharmacogenetic findings suggest that dopaminergic and serotonergic variants play a major role in the development of side effects. In particular, D2, D3 and D4 receptor variants have been clearly associated with the development of movement disorders including tardive dyskinesia (TD), akathisia and Parkinsonism during antipsychotic treatment [3, 13, 14, 36, 55, 61, 64, 72]. Additionally, there are reports of association of dopaminergic polymorphisms with weight gain, rigidity and sexual dysfunction [14, 96]. Serotonergic variants are associated to weight gain, obesity and metabolic syndrome in particular. 5-HT2C and 5-HT2A receptors are involved in the regulation of appetite and food intake, and several 5-HT2C polymorphisms are strongly associated with increase in weight during antipsychotic treatment, a finding which has been confirmed in numerous studies. 5-HT2A and 5-HT6 variants have also been linked to drug-induced weight gain, although with a moderate genetic effect [57, 59]. Several reports suggest that obesity, metabolic syndrome, TD and Parkinsonism may also be influenced by 5-HT2A and 5-HT2C [8, 14], although the associations are not so clear and their clinical utility is doubtful. Interestingly, genetic variants in adrenergic receptors type 1A and 2A (ADRA1A and ADRA2A) have only been linked to drug-induced weight gain and TD [66, 75, 78, 80], suggesting that they not play a major role in the therapeutic effects of currently available antipsychotics and contribute only to adverse reactions. Few studies have investigated the influence of neurotransmitter transporter variants on adverse reactions. Therefore, the findings of association between DAT with TD and extrapyramidal symptoms [29, 98] and of 5-HTT with weight gain and obesity [4, 98] need confirmation.

Findings in Metabolic Enzymes

Functional polymorphisms affecting the metabolic rates of drugs have been long hypothesised to contribute to adverse reactions. Pharmacogenetic research has provided evidence supporting this hypothesis. Strong associations between presence of

PM CYP2D6 variants and development of movement disorders such as TD have been reported [14]. The high plasma levels of drug metabolites associated with the presence of CYP PMs may be the cause of these associations. CYP1A2 functional variants have also been associated with TD and seizures [8, 14, 35, 54]. CYP1A2, CYP2D6 and CYP2C9 polymorphisms have also been linked to the presence of seizures, somnolence and weight gain in treated patients [24, 34, 59]. However, the clinical value of these later findings needs further investigation. Finally, MDR1 genetic variants may also be involved in the development of weight gain and movement disorders according to recent reports [19, 49].

Others

Numerous variants in genes not directly targeted by antipsychotic medications have been reported to contribute to induce ADRs. Whereas many of these findings, especially those with low genetic effects, need replication in independent studies for confirmation, the variability and plurality of function of the proteins involved may be a reflection of the complex mechanism of action of current antipsychotics. Only those findings that have been confirmed in independent studies will be mentioned in this chapter.

Several findings merit especial attention such as those linking proteins involved in the regulation of energy intake and expenditure with weight gain, obesity and other metabolic syndrome phenotypes. An initial report of association between a polymorphism in the melanocortin 4 receptor (MC4R) gene and weight gain was later confirmed in independent studies, constituting an exciting finding with putative clinical applicability [26, 27, 67]. Interestingly, this gene had been linked to obesity in the general population [85]. Furthermore, other genes involved in energy regulation, such as leptin (LEP), leptin receptor (LEPR), ghrelin (GHRL), insulin-induced gene 1 and 2 (INSIG1 and INSIG2), have also been associated with weight gain, dyslipidemia and metabolic syndrome [14, 21, 41, 42, 90]. These consistent results may contribute to the identification of subjects with genetic predisposition to increased weight during antipsychotic treatments and lead to preventive interventions. Finally, interesting associations between CNR1, RGS2, BDNF and COMT with TD, extrapyramidal symptoms (EPS) and Parkinsonism have been reported by several investigations and merit further research on their clinical utility [14, 39, 40, 52, 94] . There are many other single reports of genetic associations with weight gain and metabolic syndrome phenotypes. However, they need confirmation of their clinical value before being considered as response biomarkers.

1.2.2   Genome-Wide Association Studies (GWAS)

Genetic advances in the field of psychiatry have been boosted by the development of high-throughput methodologies such as GWAS. Although genomic strategies are relatively new in psychiatry, recent GWAS have yielded increasing and unequivocal evidence for common SNPs contributing to schizophrenia risk [44]. Unfortunately, only a limited number of GWAS have been conducted in order to explore the genetic variants involved in treatment failure or success. Difficulties in obtaining large enough samples with detailed information on response phenotypes are one of the main explanations for the lack of studies [13].

1.2.2.1 Findings Related to Antipsychotic Efficacy

To date, the largest GWA study of antipsychotic treatment outcome was performed on the CATIE sample, a cohort gathered for the investigation of antipsychotic efficacy. The cohort consisted of more than 700 patients treated with a variety of antipsychotics (olanzapine, risperidone, ziprasidone and perphenazine (FGA)) with detailed follow-up information on clinical performance [65]. Several single nucleotide polymorphisms (SNPs) in as yet unassigned genes, and in polymorphisms in ankyrin repeat and sterile a-motif domain containing 1B (*ANK1SB*), contactin-associated protein-like 5 (*CNTNAP5*) and transient receptor potential cation channel subfamily M member 1 (*TRPM1*) genes, were found to be associated with treatment efficacy [70]. Additional studies in the CATIE cohort found variants in the ETS homologous factor (*EHF*), sulfate transporter, D2, G-protein-coupled receptor 137B (*GPR137B*), carbohydrate sulfotransferase 8 (*CHST8*) and IL-1a genes associated with neurocognition improvement during treatment [69] and phosphodiesterase 4D (PDE4D), tight junction protein 1 (TJP1) and pyrophosphatase (inorganic) 2 (PPA2) genetic variants associated with the effect of antipsychotic treatment on illness severity.

A later GWA study conducted on patients treated with the antipsychotic iloperidone (*n*=457) revealed polymorphisms in the neuronal PAS domain protein 3 (*NPAS3*) and Kell blood group complex subunit-related family member 4 (*XKR4*) genes associated with treatment efficacy [60]. An interesting study integrating GWAS, transcriptomic and candidate gene approaches found variants in the *PDE7B* gene associated with response to risperidone [45]. Haloperidol response was also recently analysed by means of GWAS methodology. Two SNPs located in an intergenic region between the AT-rich interactive domain 5B (ARID5B, MRF1-like) gene and rhotekin 2 (RTKN2) gene, an intronic region located in the eukaryotic translation initiation factor 2 alpha 4 (EIF2AK4) gene, were associated with response [31].

1.2.2.2 Findings Related to Antipsychotic Side Effects

The first reported GWAS on antipsychotic response involved the investigation of drug-induced obesity in a cohort of 21 families [25]. This study identified a chromosomal region, 12q24, containing the pro-melanin-concentrating hormone (*PMCH*) gene involved in energy expenditure and food intake. A later study reported the Meis Homeobox 2 (*MEIS2*) gene associated with the effects of risperidone on hip and waist circumference [2]. The association between an MC4R polymorphism and weight gain was first observed in a GWAS conducted in patients undergoing initial exposure to SGA. This finding was later replicated in several independent candidate gene studies (see above) and constitutes one of the most significant biomarkers likely to have clinical applications.

A GWAS, conducted on a small cohort of patients ($n = 100$), revealed several genes from the gamma-aminobutyric acid (GABA) receptor pathway to be involved in drug-induced TD [46]. GWAS conducted in the CATIE cohort revealed associations between ZNF202 and PLP1 genetic variants and EPS [1]. Further analyses in the same cohort revealed genetic variants in a gene encoding for a transcription factor that controls neurogenesis (*EPF1*), in a cochaperone gene (*FIGN*) and in a neuronal specific RNA-binding protein gene (*NOVA1*) associated to Parkinsonism [5].

The majority of the susceptibility loci that have been discovered by GWAS are of small predisposing risk and therefore of limited clinical value. Additionally, the small sample sizes used in these studies recommend replication of the findings to reassess their clinical value. Nevertheless, GWAS findings have provided information on new therapeutic areas of interest that merit further research and could not have been obtained using selected gene strategies. New approaches including DNA sequencing, gene expression studies, epigenetic studies and large and prospectively assessed samples may further contribute to detect underlying genetic mechanisms [22].

1.3 Clinical Applications and Benefits of Pharmacogenetic Interventions

1.3.1 Pharmacogenetic Findings as Biomarkers of Clinical Outcome

As summarised in the previous sections, numerous genes and genetic variants have been associated with different response phenotypes. However, the lack of universal replication of findings and the confusion over the magnitude of the genetic effects observed complicate the translation of these findings into clinical practice. Table 1.3 summarises the most relevant pharmacogenetic findings and the strength of the supporting evidence, based on the number of significant reports and of the magnitude of the association. In general, the associations reported with side effects are clearer and of stronger genetic effects than associations with level of efficacy. The complexity of the response phenotype, which is determined by many genetic, clinical and environmental factors, makes it difficult to unravel the underlying causes of treatment variability. In contrast, adverse reactions are easier to determine, which facilitates the identification of underlying causes.

Of particular interest are the associations between CYP functional variants and presence of side effects. These findings are supported by the many studies linking presence of CYP mutations and plasma levels of drug metabolites [50, 51, 73, 82–84]. They constitute the most robust pharmacogenetic finding in the field of psychiatry so far [6]. It has been hypothesised that pretreatment genotyping and

Table 1.3 Summary of most significant pharmacogenetic findings

Gene	Level of efficacy	Side effects
D2	***	***
D3	**	***
5-HT2A	***	**
5-HT2C		***
CYP1A2		**
CYP2D6		***
COMT	***	**
BDNF	*	**
MC4R		***
MDR1	**	

* amount of evidence supporting the associations

subsequent dose adjustments according to the patient CYP polymorphic profile may result in a significant reduction of side effects [47]. Characterisation of CYP functional polymorphisms for dose adjustments has been successfully implemented in other medical areas such as oncology, and evidence of the clinical and economic benefits of such intervention is being gathered [37, 79]. The characterisation of MC4R, dopaminergic and serotonergic polymorphisms for the prediction of treatment-associated adverse reactions may also be of clinical interest. However, these encouraging findings require further research into their benefits before using them for the improvement of the efficacy and safety of antipsychotic treatments.

1.3.2 Pharmacogenetic Tests for Prediction of Antipsychotic Response

There are several commercial pharmacogenetic tests that provide information that may be useful for personalisation of antipsychotic treatment. Whereas many of them contain information to characterise CYP functional polymorphisms, several of them contain additional information which has not been thoroughly confirmed for the prediction of antipsychotic efficacy. Nevertheless, the use of the information provided by these tests as a prescription tool to aid in the selection of drug type and dose can have a significant impact in the improvement of clinical outcomes (Table 1.4).

To date, the only pharmacogenetic test approved by the American Food and Drug Agency (FDA) is the AmpliChip commercialised by Roche, which genotypes more than one hundred polymorphisms described in the CYP2D6 and CYP2C19 genes. This comprehensive information is useful for the dose adjustment of many antidepressant and antipsychotic medications, although several important antipsychotic metabolic pathways such as CYP1A2, CYP2C9 and CYP3A4 are not included. There are several pharmacogenetic tests (e.g. Genecept, GeneSight, Neuropharmagen) which interrogate metabolising and pharmacodynamic polymorphisms that could be used for both the selection of drug type and dose. However, several of the genes

Table 1.4 Summary of commercially available pharmacogenetic tests with application in psychiatry

Test	Genes characterised	FDA
Drug-metabolising profile		
AmpliChip	CYP2D6, CYPDC19	Yes
Drug-metabolizing profile and efficacy		
Genecept	CYP2D6, CYP2C19, 5-HTT, D2, AnkirynG, COMT, MTHFR	No
GeneSight	CYP2D6, CYP2C19, CYP2C9, CYP1A2, 5-HTT, 5-HT2A	No
Neuropharmagen	CYP1A2, CYP2D6, CYP2C9, CYP2C19, CYP3A4 and several pharmacodynamic genes	No
Side effects		
Pgxpredict	HLA	No
Hyperlipidemia array	Genes related to obesity, lipid metabolism and metabolic syndrome	No

included in these tests (e.g. 5-HTT, AnkirynG, MTHFR) have not been unequivocally proved as useful biomarkers to predict antipsychotic efficacy, and this information should be used with caution. Finally, two tests provide information that could be useful for the prediction of antipsychotic-induced side effects. Pgxpredict contains information of genetic variants in HLA genes that predicts the risk of developing severe and life-threatening agranulocytosis [15]. However, the level of prediction is far from 100 %, and therefore its use does not preclude the periodic monitoring of patients treated with neutropenia-inducing antipsychotics such as clozapine. Finally, a hyperlipidemia array containing biomarkers of obesity, hyperlipidemia and metabolic risk is under development [28].

In summary, whereas most of these tests contain useful information for the personalisation of antipsychotic treatment (e.g. characterisation of CYP functional polymorphisms), the clinical validity of other response biomarkers needs to be further confirmed before implementation.

1.4 Conclusions

Decades of pharmacogenetic research have identified several drug metabolising enzymes (CYP1A2 and CYP2D6), receptors (D2, D3, 5-HT2A, 5-HT2C and MC4R), transporters (MDR1) and schizophrenia-linked proteins (COMT and BDNF) that contribute to antipsychotic treatment variability. The genotyping of key polymorphisms in these genes may help in drug and dose selection and may increase the efficacy and safety of antipsychotic treatments. However, the use of pharmacogenetic information to assist drug selection in psychiatry is minimal. Lack of information and limited access to clinical or reference laboratories with capabilities for pharmacogenetic testing are partly to blame. However, the main reason that may hinder the use of pharmacogenetic tests is the lack of supporting research assessing the benefits. So far, no study has investigated if the adjustment of clinical doses of antipsychotics according to the patient's CYP genetic variants results in a reduction of the incidence of side effects and in an improvement of response. Similarly, no prospective study has proved that the use of pharmacogenetic prediction tests for the selection of antipsychotic positively influences the level of efficacy that is reflected in a reduction of hospitalisation time, improvement of social functioning, etc. To date, only a few studies confirm the benefits of using pharmacogenetic information to guide treatment with antidepressant medications [43]. The results of these are encouraging and show that antidepressant dose adjustment or even selection according to a few selected CYP and serotonergic variants results in a significant clinical improvement. However, no similar studies have been conducted on the benefits of pharmacogenetics on antipsychotic treatment. Therefore, there is little supporting evidence encouraging the use of pharmacogenetic information in clinical settings. Without a prospective trial to prove the clinical and economic benefits of using genetic information to aid drug and dose selection, clinicians are right to doubt the benefits of a pharmacogenetic approach. The affluence of commercial tests offering a variety of genetic information, sometimes poorly translated into clinically useful information, reinforces the need for prospective validating studies.

To conclude, pharmacogenetic research has provided evidence of the potential of using genetic information for the improvement of antipsychotic treatment in schizophrenia patients. However, before pharmacogenetic tests are widely implemented to improve the efficacy and safety of antipsychotic medications, an intermediate step including prospective trials is required to prove the clinical and economic benefits of pharmacogenetic testing. Once validated, further widespread use of pharmacogenetic testing can be achieved by introducing pharmacogenetics as part of clinicians' training, informing them of pharmacogenetics applications and benefits.

References

1. Aberg K, Adkins DE, Bukszar J, Webb BT, Caroff SN, Miller DD, Sebat J, Stroup S, Fanous AH, Vladimirov VI, Mcclay JL, Lieberman JA, Sullivan PF, Van Den Oord EJ (2010) Genomewide association study of movement-related adverse antipsychotic effects. Biol Psychiatry 67:279–282
2. Adkins DE, Aberg K, Mcclay JL, Bukszar J, Zhao Z, Jia P, Stroup TS, Perkins D, Mcevoy JP, Lieberman JA, Sullivan PF, Van Den Oord EJ (2011) Genomewide pharmacogenomic study of metabolic side effects to antipsychotic drugs. Mol Psychiatry 16:321–332
3. Al Hadithy AF, Ivanova SA, Pechlivanoglou P, Semke A, Fedorenko O, Kornetova E, Ryadovaya L, Brouwers JR, Wilffert B, Bruggeman R, Loonen AJ (2009) Tardive dyskinesia and DRD3, HTR2A and HTR2C gene polymorphisms in Russian psychiatric inpatients from Siberia. Prog Neuropsychopharmacol Biol Psychiatry 33:475–481
4. Al-janabi I, Arranz MJ, Blakemore AI, Saiz PA, Susce MT, Glaser PE, Clark D, De Leon J (2009) Association study of serotonergic gene variants with antipsychotic-induced adverse reactions. Psychiatr Genet 19:305–311
5. Alkelai A, Greenbaum L, Rigbi A, Kanyas K, Lerer B (2009) Genome-wide association study of antipsychotic-induced parkinsonism severity among schizophrenia patients. Psychopharmacology (Berl) 206:491–499

6. Altar CA, Hornberger J, Shewade A, Cruz V, Garrison J, Mrazek D (2013) Clinical validity of cytochrome P450 metabolism and serotonin gene variants in psychiatric pharmacotherapy. Int Rev Psychiatry 25:509–533
7. Anttila S, Illi A, Kampman O, Mattila KM, Lehtimäki T, Leinonen E (2004) Interaction between NOTCH4 and catechol-O-methyltransferase genotypes in schizophrenia patients with poor response to typical neuroleptics. Pharmacogenetics 14:303–307
8. Arranz MJ, De Leon J (2007) Pharmacogenetics and pharmacogenomics of schizophrenia: a review of last decade of research. Mol Psychiatry 12:707–747
9. Arranz MJ, Kapur S (2008) Pharmacogenetics in psychiatry: are we ready for widespread clinical use? Schizophr Bull 34:1130–1144
10. Arranz MJ, Munro J, Birkett J, Bolonna A, Mancama D, Sodhi M, Lesch KP, Meyer JF, Sham P, Collier DA, Murray RM, Kerwin RW (2000) Pharmacogenetic prediction of clozapine response. Lancet 355:1615–1616
11. Arranz MJ, Munro J, Osborne S, Collier D, Kerwin RW (2000) Difficulties in replication of results. Lancet 356:1359–1360
12. Arranz MJ, Munro J, Sham P, Kirov G, Murray RM, Collier DA, Kerwin RW (1998) Meta-analysis of studies on genetic variation in 5-HT2A receptors and clozapine response. Schizophr Res 32:93–99
13. Arranz MJ, Munro JC (2011) Toward understanding genetic risk for differential antipsychotic response in individuals with schizophrenia. Expert Rev Clin Pharmacol 4:389–405
14. Arranz MJ, Rivera M, Munro JC (2011) Pharmacogenetics of response to antipsychotics in patients with schizophrenia. CNS Drugs 25:933–969
15. Athanasiou MC, Dettling M, Cascorbi I, Mosyagin I, Salisbury BA, Pierz KA, Zou W, Whalen H, Malhotra AK, Lencz T, Gerson SL, Kane JM, Reed CR (2011) Candidate gene analysis identifies a polymorphism in HLA-DQB1 associated with clozapine-induced agranulocytosis. J Clin Psychiatry 72:458–463
16. Bertolino A, Caforio G, Blasi G, Rampino A, Nardini M, Weinberger DR, Dallapiccola B, Sinibaldi L, Douzgou S (2007) COMT Val158Met polymorphism predicts negative symptoms response to treatment with olanzapine in schizophrenia. Schizophr Res 95:253–255
17. Bilic P, Jukic V, Vilibic M, Savic A, Bozina N (2014) Treatment-resistant schizophrenia and DAT and SERT polymorphisms. Gene 543:125–132
18. Bondolfi G, Morel F, Crettol S, Rachid F, Baumann P, Eap CB (2005) Increased clozapine plasma concentrations and side effects induced by smoking cessation in 2 CYP1A2 genotyped patients. Ther Drug Monit 27:539–543
19. Bozina N, Kuzman MR, Medved V, Jovanovic N, Sertic J, Hotujac L (2008) Associations between MDR1 gene polymorphisms and schizophrenia and therapeutic response to olanzapine in female schizophrenic patients. J Psychiatr Res 42:89–97
20. Bozina N, Medved V, Kuzman MR, Sain I, Sertic J (2007) Association study of olanzapine-induced weight gain and therapeutic response with SERT gene polymorphisms in female schizophrenic patients. J Psychopharmacol 21:728–734
21. Brandl EJ, Frydrychowicz C, Tiwari AK, Lett TA, Kitzrow W, Büttner S, Ehrlich S, Meltzer HY, Lieberman JA, Kennedy JL, Müller DJ, Puls I (2012) Association study of polymorphisms in leptin and leptin receptor genes with antipsychotic-induced body weight gain. Prog Neuropsychopharmacol Biol Psychiatry 38:134–141
22. Brandl EJ, Kennedy JL, Muller DJ (2014) Pharmacogenetics of antipsychotics. Can J Psychiatry 59:76–88
23. Brockmöller J, Kirchheiner J, Schmider J, Walter S, Sachse C, Müller-oerlinghausen B, Roots I (2002) The impact of the CYP2D6 polymorphism on haloperidol pharmacokinetics and on the outcome of haloperidol treatment. Clin Pharmacol Ther 72:438–452
24. Cabaleiro T, López-rodríguez R, Román M, Ochoa D, Novalbos J, Borobia A, Carcas A, Abad-santos F (2015) Pharmacogenetics of quetiapine in healthy volunteers: association with pharmacokinetics, pharmacodynamics, and adverse effects. Int Clin Psychopharmacol 30:82–88

25. Chagnon YC, Merette C, Bouchard RH, Emond C, Roy MA, Maziade M (2004) A genome wide linkage study of obesity as secondary effect of antipsychotics in multigenerational families of eastern Quebec affected by psychoses. Mol Psychiatry 9:1067–1074
26. Chowdhury NI, Tiwari AK, Souza RP, Zai CC, Shaikh SA, Chen S, Liu F, Lieberman JA, Meltzer HY, Malhotra AK, Kennedy JL, Müller DJ (2013) Genetic association study between antipsychotic-induced weight gain and the melanocortin-4 receptor gene. Pharmacogenomics J 13:272–279
27. Czerwensky F, Leucht S, Steimer W (2013) MC4R rs489693: a clinical risk factor for second generation antipsychotic-related weight gain? Int J Neuropsychopharmacol 16:2103–2109
28. De Leon J, Correa JC, Ruaño G, Windemuth A, Arranz MJ, Diaz FJ (2008) Exploring genetic variations that may be associated with the direct effects of some antipsychotics on lipid levels. Schizophr Res 98:40–46
29. De Leon J, Susce MT, Pan RM, Koch WH, Wedlund PJ (2005) Polymorphic variations in GSTM1, GSTT1, PgP, CYP2D6, CYP3A5, and dopamine D2 and D3 receptors and their association with tardive dyskinesia in severe mental illness. J Clin Psychopharmacol 25:448–456
30. De Vos A, Van Der Weide J, Loovers HM (2011) Association between CYP2C19*17 and metabolism of amitriptyline, citalopram and clomipramine in Dutch hospitalized patients. Pharmacogenomics J 11:359–367
31. Drago A, Giegling I, Schafer M, Hartmann AM, Konte B, Friedl M, Serretti A, Rujescu D (2014) Genome-wide association study supports the role of the immunological system and of the neurodevelopmental processes in response to haloperidol treatment. Pharmacogenet Genomics 24:314–319
32. Du J, Zhang A, Wang L, Xuan J, Yu L, Che R, Li X, Gu N, Lin Z, Feng G, Xing Q, He L (2010) Relationship between response to risperidone, plasma concentrations of risperidone and CYP3A4 polymorphisms in schizophrenia patients. J Psychopharmacol 24:1115–1120
33. Eap CB, Bender S, Jaquenoud Sirot E, Cucchia G, Jonzier-Perey M, Baumann P, Allorge D, Broly F (2004) Nonresponse to clozapine and ultrarapid CYP1A2 activity: clinical data and analysis of CYP1A2 gene. J Clin Psychopharmacol 24:214–219
34. Ellingrod VL, Miller D, Schultz SK, Wehring H, Arndt S (2002) CYP2D6 polymorphisms and atypical antipsychotic weight gain. Psychiatr Genet 12:55–58
35. Ferrari M, Bolla E, Bortolaso P, Callegari C, Poloni N, Lecchini S, Vender S, Marino F, Cosentino M (2012) Association between CYP1A2 polymorphisms and clozapine-induced adverse reactions in patients with schizophrenia. Psychiatry Res 200:1014–1017
36. Fijal BA, Kohler J, Ostbye K, Ahl J, Houston JP (2013) Association of candidate gene polymorphisms with diastolic blood pressure change in patients treated with duloxetine. Psychiatry Res 206:313–314
37. Fleeman N, Martin Saborido C, Payne K, Boland A, Dickson R, Dundar Y, Fernández santander A, Howell S, Newman W, Oyee J, Walley T (2011) The clinical effectiveness and cost-effectiveness of genotyping for CYP2D6 for the management of women with breast cancer treated with tamoxifen: a systematic review. Health Technol Assess 15:1–102
38. Fleeman N, Mcleod C, Bagust A, Beale S, Boland A, Dundar Y, Jorgensen A, Payne K, Pirmohamed M, Pushpakom S, Walley T, De Warren-Penny P, Dickson R (2010) The clinical effectiveness and cost-effectiveness of testing for cytochrome P450 polymorphisms in patients with schizophrenia treated with antipsychotics: a systematic review and economic evaluation. Health Technol Assess 14:1–157, iii
39. Gareeva AE, Zakirov DF, Valinurov RG, Khusnutdinova EK (2013) Polymorphism of RGS2 gene: genetic markers of risk for schizophrenia and pharmacogenetic markers of typical neuroleptics efficiency. Mol Biol (Mosk) 47:934–941
40. Greenbaum L, Alkelai A, Zozulinsky P, Kohn Y, Lerer B (2012) Support for association of HSPG2 with tardive dyskinesia in Caucasian populations. Pharmacogenomics J 12:513–520
41. Gregoor JG, Van Der Weide J, Loovers HM, VAN Megen HJ, Egberts TC, Heerdink ER (2011) Polymorphisms of the LEP, LEPR and HTR2C gene: obesity and BMI change in patients using antipsychotic medication in a naturalistic setting. Pharmacogenomics 12:919–923

42. Gregoor JG, Van Der Weide J, Mulder H, Cohen D, Van Megen HJ, Egberts AC, Heerdink ER (2009) Polymorphisms of the LEP- and LEPR gene and obesity in patients using antipsychotic medication. J Clin Psychopharmacol 29:21–25

43. Hall-Flavin DK, Winner JG, Allen JD, Jordan JJ, Nesheim RS, Snyder KA, Drews MS, Eisterhold LL, Biernacka JM, Mrazek DA (2012) Using a pharmacogenomic algorithm to guide the treatment of depression. Transl Psychiatry 2, e172

44. Harrison PJ (2015) Recent genetic findings in schizophrenia and their therapeutic relevance. J Psychopharmacol 29:85–96

45. Ikeda M, Tomita Y, Mouri A, Koga M, Okochi T, Yoshimura R, Yamanouchi Y, Kinoshita Y, Hashimoto R, Williams HJ, Takeda M, Nakamura J, Nabeshima T, Owen MJ, O'donovan MC, Honda H, Arinami T, Ozaki N, Iwata N (2010) Identification of novel candidate genes for treatment response to risperidone and susceptibility for schizophrenia: integrated analysis among pharmacogenomics, mouse expression, and genetic case–control association approaches. Biol Psychiatry 67:263–269

46. Inada T, Koga M, Ishiguro H, Horiuchi Y, Syu A, Yoshio T, Takahashi N, Ozaki N, Arinami T (2008) Pathway-based association analysis of genome-wide screening data suggest that genes associated with the gamma-aminobutyric acid receptor signaling pathway are involved in neuroleptic-induced, treatment-resistant tardive dyskinesia. Pharmacogenet Genomics 18: 317–323

47. Ingelman-Sundberg M (2004) Pharmacogenetics of cytochrome P450 and its applications in drug therapy: the past, present and future. Trends Pharmacol Sci 25:193–200

48. Joober R, Benkelfat C, Lal S, Bloom D, Labelle A, Lalonde P, Turecki G, Rozen R, Rouleau GA (2000) Association between the methylenetetrahydrofolate reductase 677C-->T missense mutation and schizophrenia. Mol Psychiatry 5:323–326

49. Kastelic M, Koprivsek J, Plesnicar BK, Serretti A, Mandelli L, Locatelli I, Grabnar I, Dolzan V (2010) MDR1 gene polymorphisms and response to acute risperidone treatment. Prog Neuropsychopharmacol Biol Psychiatry 34:387–392

50. Kingbäck M, Karlsson L, Zackrisson AL, Carlsson B, Josefsson M, Bengtsson F, Ahlner J, Kugelberg FC (2012) Influence of CYP2D6 genotype on the disposition of the enantiomers of venlafaxine and its major metabolites in postmortem femoral blood. Forensic Sci Int 214: 124–134

51. Kirchheiner J, Meineke I, Müller G, Bauer S, Rohde W, Meisel C, Roots I, Brockmöller J (2004) Influence of CYP2C9 and CYP2D6 polymorphisms on the pharmacokinetics of nateglinide in genotyped healthy volunteers. Clin Pharmacokinet 43:267–278

52. Knol W, Van Marum RJ, Jansen PA, Strengman E, Al Hadithy AF, Wilffert B, Schobben AA, Ophoff RA, Egberts TC (2013) Genetic variation and the risk of haloperidol-related parkinsonism in elderly patients: a candidate gene approach. J Clin Psychopharmacol 33:405–410

53. Kohlrausch FB, Salatino-Oliveira A, Gama CS, Lobato MI, Belmonte-De-Abreu P, Hutz MH (2010) Influence of serotonin transporter gene polymorphisms on clozapine response in Brazilian schizophrenics. J Psychiatr Res 44:1158–1162

54. Kohlrausch FB, Severino-Gama C, Lobato MI, Belmonte-De-Abreu P, Carracedo A, Hutz MH (2013) The CYP1A2 -163C>A polymorphism is associated with clozapine-induced generalized tonic-clonic seizures in Brazilian schizophrenia patients. Psychiatry Res 209:242–245

55. Koning JP, Vehof J, Burger H, Wilffert B, Al Hadithy A, Alizadeh B, Van Harten PN, Snieder H, Genetic Risk and Outcome in Psychosis (GROUP) investigators (2012) Association of two DRD2 gene polymorphisms with acute and tardive antipsychotic-induced movement disorders in young Caucasian patients. Psychopharmacology (Berl) 219:727–736

56. Krebs MO, Guillin O, Bourdell MC, Schwartz JC, Olie JP, Poirier MF, Sokoloff P (2000) Brain derived neurotrophic factor (BDNF) gene variants association with age at onset and therapeutic response in schizophrenia. Mol Psychiatry 5:558–562

57. Lane HY, Lin CC, Huang CH, Chang YC, Hsu SK, Chang WH (2004) Risperidone response and 5-HT6 receptor gene variance: genetic association analysis with adjustment for nongenetic confounders. Schizophr Res 67:63–70

58. Lane HY, Liu YC, Huang CL, Chang YC, Wu PL, Huang CH, Tsai GE (2008) RGS4 polymorphisms predict clinical manifestations and responses to risperidone treatment in patients with schizophrenia. J Clin Psychopharmacol 28:64–68
59. Lane HY, Liu YC, Huang CL, Chang YC, Wu PL, Lu CT, Chang WH (2006) Risperidone-related weight gain: genetic and nongenetic predictors. J Clin Psychopharmacol 26:128–134
60. Lavedan C, Licamele L, Volpi S, Hamilton J, Heaton C, Mack K, Lannan R, Thompson A, Wolfgang CD, Polymeropoulos MH (2009) Association of the NPAS3 gene and five other loci with response to the antipsychotic iloperidone identified in a whole genome association study. Mol Psychiatry 14:804–819
61. Lawford BR, Barnes M, Swagell CD, Connor JP, Burton SC, Heslop K, Voisey J, Morris CP, Nyst P, Noble EP, Young RM (2013) DRD2/ANKK1 Taq1A (rs 1800497 C>T) genotypes are associated with susceptibility to second generation antipsychotic-induced akathisia. J Psychopharmacol 27:343–348
62. Lee ST, Ryu S, Kim SR, Kim MJ, Kim S, Kim JW, Lee SY, Hong KS (2012) Association study of 27 annotated genes for clozapine pharmacogenetics: validation of preexisting studies and identification of a new candidate gene, ABCB1, for treatment response. J Clin Psychopharmacol 32:441–448
63. Leon J, Susce MT, Pan RM, Wedlund PJ, Orrego ML, Diaz FJ (2007) A study of genetic (CYP2D6 and ABCB1) and environmental (drug inhibitors and inducers) variables that may influence plasma risperidone levels. Pharmacopsychiatry 40:93–102
64. Lerer B, Segman RH, Fangerau H, Daly AK, Basile VS, Cavallaro R, Aschauer HN, Mccreadie RG, Ohlraun S, Ferrier N, Masellis M, Verga M, Scharfetter J, Rietschel M, Lovlie R, Levy UH, Meltzer HY, Kennedy JL, Steen VM, Macciardi F (2002) Pharmacogenetics of tardive dyskinesia: combined analysis of 780 patients supports association with dopamine D3 receptor gene Ser9Gly polymorphism. Neuropsychopharmacology 27:105–119
65. Lieberman JA, Stroup TS, Mcevoy JP, Swartz MS, Rosenheck RA, Perkins DO, Keefe RS, Davis SM, Davis CE, Lebowitz BD, Severe J, Hsiao JK (2005) Effectiveness of antipsychotic drugs in patients with chronic schizophrenia. N Engl J Med 353:1209–1223
66. Liu YR, Loh EW, Lan TH, Chen SF, Yu YH, Chang YH, Huang CJ, Hu TM, Lin KM, Yao YT, Chiu HJ (2010) ADRA1A gene is associated with BMI in chronic schizophrenia patients exposed to antipsychotics. Pharmacogenomics J 10:30–39
67. Malhotra AK, Correll CU, Chowdhury NI, Müller DJ, Gregersen PK, Lee AT, Tiwari AK, Kane JM, Fleischhacker WW, Kahn RS, Ophoff RA, Meltzer HY, Lencz T, Kennedy JL (2012) Association between common variants near the melanocortin 4 receptor gene and severe antipsychotic drug-induced weight gain. Arch Gen Psychiatry 69:904–912
68. Mancama D, Arranz MJ, Munro J, Osborne S, Makoff A, Collier D, Kerwin R (2002) Investigation of promoter variants of the histamine 1 and 2 receptors in schizophrenia and clozapine response. Neurosci Lett 333:207–211
69. Mcclay JL, Adkins DE, Aberg K, Bukszar J, Khachane AN, Keefe RS, Perkins DO, Mcevoy JP, Stroup TS, Vann RE, Beardsley PM, Lieberman JA, Sullivan PF, Van Den Oord EJ (2011) Genome-wide pharmacogenomic study of neurocognition as an indicator of antipsychotic treatment response in schizophrenia. Neuropsychopharmacology 36:616–626
70. Mcclay JL, Adkins DE, Aberg K, Stroup S, Perkins DO, Vladimirov VI, Lieberman JA, Sullivan PF, Van Den Oord EJ (2011) Genome-wide pharmacogenomic analysis of response to treatment with antipsychotics. Mol Psychiatry 16:76–85
71. Molero P, Ortuño F, Zalacain M, Patiño-García A (2007) Clinical involvement of catechol-O-methyltransferase polymorphisms in schizophrenia spectrum disorders: influence on the severity of psychotic symptoms and on the response to neuroleptic treatment. Pharmacogenomics J 7:418–426
72. Müller DJ, Zai CC, Sicard M, Remington E, Souza RP, Tiwari AK, Hwang R, Likhodi O, Shaikh S, Freeman N, Arenovich T, Heinz A, Meltzer HY, Lieberman JA, Kennedy JL (2012) Systematic analysis of dopamine receptor genes (DRD1-DRD5) in antipsychotic-induced weight gain. Pharmacogenomics J 12:156–164

73. Nikisch G, baumann P, Oneda B, Kiessling B, Weisser H, Mathé AA, Yoshitake T, Kehr J, Wiedemann G, Eap CB (2011) Cytochrome P450 and ABCB1 genetics: association with quetiapine and norquetiapine plasma and cerebrospinal fluid concentrations and with clinical response in patients suffering from schizophrenia. A pilot study. J Psychopharmacol 25: 896–907

74. Ota VK, Spíndola LN, Gadelha A, Dos Santos Filho AF, Santoro ML, Christofolini DM, Bellucco FT, Ribeiro-Dos-Santos Â, Santos S, Mari JEJ, Melaragno MI, Bressan RA, Smith MEA, Belangero SI (2012) DRD1 rs4532 polymorphism: a potential pharmacogenomic marker for treatment response to antipsychotic drugs. Schizophr Res 142:206–208

75. Park YM, Chung YC, Lee SH, Lee KJ, Kim H, Byun YC, Lim SW, Paik JW, Lee HJ (2006) Weight gain associated with the alpha2a-adrenergic receptor −1,291 C/G polymorphism and olanzapine treatment. Am J Med Genet B Neuropsychiatr Genet 141B:394–397

76. Rajkumar AP, Poonkuzhali B, Kuruvilla A, Srivastava A, Jacob M, Jacob KS (2012) Outcome definitions and clinical predictors influence pharmacogenetic associations between HTR3A gene polymorphisms and response to clozapine in patients with schizophrenia. Psychopharmacology (Berl) 224:441–449

77. Rau T, Wohlleben G, Wuttke H, Thuerauf N, Lunkenheimer J, Lanczik M, Eschenhagen T (2004) CYP2D6 genotype: impact on adverse effects and nonresponse during treatment with antidepressants-a pilot study. Clin Pharmacol Ther 75:386–393

78. Saiz PA, Susce MT, Clark DA, Kerwin RW, Molero P, Arranz MJ, De Leon J (2008) An investigation of the alpha1A-adrenergic receptor gene and antipsychotic-induced side-effects. Hum Psychopharmacol 23:107–114

79. Schroth W, Hamann U, Fasching PA, Dauser S, Winter S, Eichelbaum M, Schwab M, Brauch H (2010) CYP2D6 polymorphisms as predictors of outcome in breast cancer patients treated with tamoxifen: expanded polymorphism coverage improves risk stratification. Clin Cancer Res 16:4468–4477

80. Sickert L, Müller DJ, Tiwari AK, Shaikh S, Zai C, DE Souza R, De Luca V, Meltzer HY, Lieberman JA, Kennedy JL (2009) Association of the alpha 2A adrenergic receptor -1291C/G polymorphism and antipsychotic-induced weight gain in European-Americans. Pharmacogenomics 10:1169–1176

81. Suzuki T, Mihara K, Nakamura A, Nagai G, Kagawa S, Nemoto K, Ohta I, Arakaki H, Uno T, Kondo T (2011) Effects of the CYP2D6*10 allele on the steady-state plasma concentrations of aripiprazole and its active metabolite, dehydroaripiprazole, in Japanese patients with schizophrenia. Ther Drug Monit 33:21–24

82. Suzuki Y, Fukui N, Tsuneyama N, Watanabe J, Ono S, Sugai T, Saito M, Inoue Y, Someya T (2012) Effect of the cytochrome P450 2D6*10 allele on risperidone metabolism in Japanese psychiatric patients. Hum Psychopharmacol 27:43–46

83. Tsai MH, Lin KM, Hsiao MC, Shen WW, Lu ML, Tang HS, Fang CK, Wu CS, Lu SC, Liu SC, Chen CY, Liu YL (2010) Genetic polymorphisms of cytochrome P450 enzymes influence metabolism of the antidepressant escitalopram and treatment response. Pharmacogenomics 11:537–546

84. van der Weide J, van Baalen-Benedek EH, Kootstra-Ros JE (2005) Metabolic ratios of psychotropics as indication of cytochrome P450 2D6/2C19 genotype. Ther Drug Monit 27:478–483

85. Wang J, Mei H, Chen W, Jiang Y, Sun W, Li F, Fu Q, Jiang F (2012) Study of eight GWAS-identified common variants for association with obesity-related indices in Chinese children at puberty. Int J Obes (Lond) 36:542–547

86. Wang L, Yu L, He G, Zhang J, Zhang AP, Du J, Tang RQ, Zhao XZ, Ma J, Xuan JK, Xiao Y, Gu NF, Feng GY, Xu MQ, Xing QH, He L (2007) Response of risperidone treatment may be associated with polymorphisms of HTT gene in Chinese schizophrenia patients. Neurosci Lett 414:1–4

87. Wei Z, Wang L, Yu T, Wang Y, Sun L, Wang T, Huo R, Li Y, Wu X, Qin S, Xu Y, Feng G, He L, Xing Q (2013) Histamine H4 receptor polymorphism: a potential predictor of risperidone efficacy. J Clin Psychopharmacol 33:221–225

88. Wei Z, Wang L, Zhang M, Xuan J, Wang Y, Liu B, Shao L, Li J, Zeng Z, Li T, Liu J, Wang T, Qin S, Xu Y, Feng G, He L, Xing Q (2012) A pharmacogenetic study of risperidone on histamine H3 receptor gene (HRH3) in Chinese Han schizophrenia patients. J Psychopharmacol 26:813–818
89. Weickert TW, Goldberg TE, Mishara A, Apud JA, Kolachana BS, Egan MF, Weinberger DR (2004) Catechol-O-methyltransferase val108/158met genotype predicts working memory response to antipsychotic medications. Biol Psychiatry 56:677–682
90. Wu R, Zhao J, Shao P, Ou J, Chang M (2011) Genetic predictors of antipsychotic-induced weight gain: a case-matched multi-gene study. Zhong Nan Da Xue Xue Bao Yi Xue Ban 36:720–723
91. Xiang Q, Zhao X, Zhou Y, Duan JL, Cui YM (2010) Effect of CYP2D6, CYP3A5, and MDR1 genetic polymorphisms on the pharmacokinetics of risperidone and its active moiety. J Clin Pharmacol 50:659–666
92. Xing Q, Gao R, Li H, Feng G, Xu M, Duan S, Meng J, Zhang A, Qin S, He L (2006) Polymorphisms of the ABCB1 gene are associated with the therapeutic response to risperidone in Chinese schizophrenia patients. Pharmacogenomics 7:987–993
93. Yasui-Furukori N, Saito M, Nakagami T, Kaneda A, Tateishi T, Kaneko S (2006) Association between multidrug resistance 1 (MDR1) gene polymorphisms and therapeutic response to bromperidol in schizophrenic patients: a preliminary study. Prog Neuropsychopharmacol Biol Psychiatry 30:286–291
94. Zai GC, Zai CC, Chowdhury NI, Tiwari AK, Souza RP, Lieberman JA, Meltzer HY, Potkin SG, Müller DJ, Kennedy JL (2012) The role of brain-derived neurotrophic factor (BDNF) gene variants in antipsychotic response and antipsychotic-induced weight gain. Prog Neuropsychopharmacol Biol Psychiatry 39:96–101
95. Zhang JP, Lencz T, Geisler S, Derosse P, Bromet EJ, Malhotra AK (2013) Genetic variation in BDNF is associated with antipsychotic treatment resistance in patients with schizophrenia. Schizophr Res 146:285–288
96. Zhang XR, Zhang ZJ, Zhu RX, Yuan YG, Jenkins TA, Reynolds GP (2011) Sexual dysfunction in male schizophrenia: influence of antipsychotic drugs, prolactin and polymorphisms of the dopamine D2 receptor genes. Pharmacogenomics 12:1127–1136
97. Zhao QZ, Liu BC, Zhang J, Wang L, Li XW, Wang Y, Ji J, Yang FP, Wan CL, Xu YF, Feng GY, He L, He G (2012) Association between a COMT polymorphism and clinical response to risperidone treatment: a pharmacogenetic study. Psychiatr Genet 22:298–299
98. Zivković M, Mihaljević-Peles A, Bozina N, Sagud M, Nikolac-Perkovic M, Vuksan-Cusa B, Muck-Seler D (2013) The association study of polymorphisms in DAT, DRD2, and COMT genes and acute extrapyramidal adverse effects in male schizophrenic patients treated with haloperidol. J Clin Psychopharmacol 33:593–599

Chapter 2
Pharmacogenetics of Serious Antipsychotic Side Effects

Malgorzata Maciukiewicz, Venuja Sriretnakumar, and Daniel J. Müller

Abstract First- and second-generation antipsychotics are common drugs for treatment of schizophrenia (SCZ). Both classes of drugs have different receptor-binding profiles and affinities that are likely involved in their propensity to cause adverse side effects such as tardive dyskinesia (TD), antipsychotic-induced weight gain (AIWG) and clozapine-induced agranulocytosis (CIA). Apart from clinical and demographic factors (e.g. age, drug exposure, etc.) associated with risk for specific antipsychotic-induced side effects, genetic factors have also been shown to modulate outcome to antispychotic drugs. Notably, some of the studied genetic variants have been shown to have relatively large effect sizes in the risk for specific side effects. Beyond genes involved in drug metabolism (in particular *CYP2D6* and *CYP1A2*), *SLC18A2*, *PIP5K2A*, *CNR1*, *DPP6* and *HSPG2* gene variants have more recently been found to be associated with TD. Similarly, *HTR2C*, *LEP*, *MC4R*, *NDUFS1* and *CNR1* genes have been associated with AIWG in at least two independent samples. Finally, variants of the HLA and MPO genes have been associated with CIA. Notably, the first genetic test kits designed to reduce risk of antipsychotic-induced side effects have become available for use in clinical practice. However, the clinical relevance of these gene variants needs further evaluation, and future studies are required to better understand the molecular context of the variants in these side effects.

M. Maciukiewicz
Pharmacogenetics Research Clinic, Campbell Family Mental Health Research Institute,
Centre for Addiction and Mental Health, Toronto, ON, Canada

V. Sriretnakumar
Pharmacogenetics Research Clinic, Campbell Family Mental Health Research Institute,
Centre for Addiction and Mental Health, Toronto, ON, Canada

Department of Laboratory Medicine and Pathobiology, University of Toronto,
Toronto, ON, Canada

D.J. Müller, MD, PhD (✉)
Pharmacogenetics Research Clinic, Campbell Family Mental Health Research Institute,
Centre for Addiction and Mental Health, Toronto, ON, Canada

Institute of Medical Science, Faculty of Medicine, University of Toronto,
Toronto, ON, Canada

Department of Psychiatry, University of Toronto, Toronto, ON, Canada
e-mail: daniel.mueller@camh.ca

© Springer International Publishing Switzerland 2016
J.K. Rybakowski, A. Serretti (eds.), *Genetic Influences on Response to Drug Treatment for Major Psychiatric Disorders*, DOI 10.1007/978-3-319-27040-1_2

2.1 Background

Antipsychotic (AP) drugs are widely used in the treatment of various psychiatric disorders, including schizophrenia (SCZ), bipolar disorders (BD) and autism. Traditionally, AP drugs are divided into two classes: first-generation APs (FGAPs, also known as typical antipsychotics) and second-generation APs (SGAPs, commonly known as atypical antipsychotics).

AP drugs can be quite effective in treating the debilitating clinical symptoms in many psychiatric disorders. However, despite APs' clinical efficacy, they are also associated with various and serious adverse side effects in AP-treated patients. Extrapyramidal effects (EPS), such as tardive dyskinesia (TD), are severe movement disorders primarily associated with FGAPs. The side effects of FGAPs can be acute (e.g. dystonia, akathisia) or chronic (e.g. TD) [58]. Movement disturbances can present itself during SGAPs; however, it is a less common occurrence [77]. The main adverse effects of SGAPs are antipsychotic-induced weight gain (AIWG) and associated metabolic dysregulation, leading to type II diabetes and cardiovascular diseases [50]. Moreover, clozapine is an important SGAP that is specifically used in the treatment of SCZ refractory patients. Regardless of clozapine's efficacy in treatment-resistance SCZ patients, it has been associated with the development of potentially fatal agranulocytosis, along with the more common SGAP side effects (e.g. AIWG) [75]. Put together, the adverse drug reactions of APs presents a significant clinical challenge in the treatment of SCZ patients.

The high variability in AP treatment response amongst individuals results in a trial-and-error practice of various prescriptions before a suitable medication for a patient is identified. Many variables contribute to inter-individual differences in treatment response and risk for side effects including age, diet, smoking, exposure to previous and concurrent medications, disease severity, and most importantly, genetic factors. While many different side effects have been associated with AP treatment, previous genetic studies have predominantly focused on TD, AIWG, and clozapine-induced agranulocytosis (CIA). Therefore, this chapter will focus on these common and serious side effects, providing a concise summary of the genetic associations found thus far in the scientific literature. We included studies that describe gene variants reported in at least two independent samples or through genome-wide association studies (GWAS).

2.2 Common Side Effects

2.2.1 Tardive Dyskinesia

Tardive dyskinesia (TD) is a severe side effect characterised by involuntary trunk, limb, and orofacial muscle movements, it is found to be present in 20–30 % of patients treated with FGAPs [33]. Family studies have shown a strong genetic component for TD risk [61]. The pathophysiology of TD is not yet fully understood, however, several molecular pathways have been implicated [47]. Based on these observations, substantial efforts have been made through candidate gene studies and GWAS to identify risk variants associated with the development of TD in FGAP-treated SCZ patients.

2.2.1.1 Drug Metabolism Genes

Cytochrome P450 (*CYP*) genes have many functions, including the regulation of oxidative stress and the clearance of drugs in the liver [14]. In particular, *CYP2D6* and *CYP1A2* genes code for enzymes crucial for the metabolism of most AP drugs [60]. Interestingly, *CYP2D6* is also expressed in the brain, where it is involved in the metabolism of intrinsic agents, such as neurotransmitters metabolites, which may play a role in the development of TD [14]. *CYP2D6* is a highly polymorphic gene with more than 100 variants discovered to date [24]. Such variants may alter the encoding protein functions resulting in either increased or decreased enzyme activity, consequently altering drug metabolism [24].

Genetic association studies between *CYP* variants and TD have produced mixed results [53]. One meta-analysis study has linked loss of function in *CYP2D6* to TD [66], whereas recent findings suggest that ultra-rapid *CYP2D6* metabolizers, with increased enzyme activity, are at a higher risk for TD [44]. This finding implies higher serum concentrations of the AP drug metabolites, due to rapid conversion of drug into their metabolites, as a risk factor for TD in ultra-rapid metabolizers. *CYP2D6* now undergoes growing interest as potential tardive dyskinesia genetic risk marker.

FGAPs such as haloperidol are metabolised mainly by *CYP1A2* enzyme [5]. The C allele of *CYP1A2* was significantly more frequent in cases with TD when compared with controls [23, 83]. A recent study on a Russian sample showed that the CC genotype was linked with higher severity of TD [32]; however, results were not significant following correction for age and gender. *CYP1A2* variants are promising candidates for TD genetic testing; however, more replication studies are required to confirm the association of *CYP1A2* variant in relation to TD.

2.2.1.2 Neurotransmitter Genes

APs modulate a variety of neurotransmitter receptors, mainly dopamine, serotonin, adrenergic, glutamate, and histamine receptors [47]. Several genetic association studies have been conducted between genes related with neurotransmitter pathways, in particular dopamine (*DRD2, DRD3* and *DRD4*), and serotonin receptors (*5-HT2A, HTR3A*).

Dopamine System Genes

It is hypothesised that dopamine hypersensitivity might lead to TD occurrence in SCZ patients [69]. FGAPs, characterised by high affinity to dopamine D2 receptors, are known to cause EPS symptoms, including TD [40]. On the other hand, SGAPs, such as clozapine and olanzapine, show lower dopamine D2 affinity and lower risk for EPS symptoms [39].

The *TaqIA* (rs1800497) variant of the dopamine D2 receptor (*DRD2*) gene locus has been extensively studied amongst different populations, albeit with mixed results. A meta-analysis from 2007 showed *TaqIA* A2 allele and A2/A2 genotype to be risk factors for TD [97]. A more recent study has shown association between *TaqIA* and TD in Caucasians [43]. However, another study has not supported this finding in a Korean population [65].

Genetic association studies of the variant of the dopamine D3 receptor (*DRD3*) have also provided mixed results amongst the literature. Three independent studies have found the Ser9Gly variant to be a risk factor of TD in the Caucasian population [2, 51, 71]. Despite previous findings, two recent meta-analyses have not been able to replicate the association between the Ser9Gly variant and TD [89, 92]. Similar to the *TaqIA* variant, the mixed results for Ser9Gly and TD could be due to population stratification effects.

The vesicular monoamine transporter 2 (*SLC18A2*) variant rs2015586 has been studied as part of a large pharmacogenetic investigation of TD in SCZ [88]. This candidate gene study found rs2015586 to be significantly associated with TD prior to correction for multiple testing [88]. Recent analysis has confirmed that *SLC18A2* C allele could be a risk variant of TD. Additionally, significant interaction between the DRD2 rs6277 and SLC18A2 rs363224 markers have been discovered [99].

Dopamine system genes may play a role in tardive dyskinesia. More research, across different ethnic groups, is needed to elucidate their associations with TD.

Serotonin System Genes

SGAPs such as olanzapine and clozapine are characterised by higher serotonin receptor affinities and are known to have a lower risk for TD compared to FGAPs [56].

5-HT2A serotonin receptors, present in the basal ganglia, play a significant role in the development of movement disorders [47]. One study has found associations between the T102C (rs6313) variant of the serotonin 2A receptor gene (*HTR2A*) and TD in a mixed ancestry sample [49]. This association has been later replicated in a Taiwanese sample [31]. This gene can be a good candidate for screening individuals for TD risk, especially since this variant showed the same effect across different ethnic groups.

Two recent studies have investigated associations between *HTR2C* serotonin receptor variants and TD [3, 43]. An association between *HTR2C* rs4911871 variant and orofacial dyskinesia has been found. The rs4911871 may be a promising candidate for genetic screening; however, more studies are required.

2.2.1.3 Oxidative Stress Genes

Oxidative stress and the resultant reactive oxygen species (ROS) are suggested to cause neuronal degeneration and contribute to TD. Neuronal cells have been shown to be highly sensitive and prone to oxidative damage [47]. Thus, conferring oxidative stress and antioxidant pathway-related genes have been described as promising candidates for genetic studies of TD.

One such candidate gene is the mitochondrial enzyme manganese superoxide dismutase (*MnSOD*). *MnSOD* is part of the antioxidant pathway responsible for neutralising superoxide anions and has been analysed in multiple genetic association studies, albeit with conflicting results. Two meta-analyses have been conducted thus far to assess the effect of Ala-9Val *MnSOD* variant in TD. Results to date suggests a protective effect of the Val allele; however, a recent meta-analysis has found no effect of Ala-9Val on TD [98]. Studies following the meta-analysis by Zai et al. [98] suggested an association of the Val/Val genotype with negative symptoms in SCZ, but not TD, in a Chinese cohort [52]. A more recent analysis however has not confirmed a major role of Ala-9Val variant in EPS development [6]. In summary, genetic association studies of *MnSOD* and its Ala-9Val variant provided mixed results; thus it is unlikely that the *MnSOD* gene plays a major role in TD.

The phosphatidylinositol-5-phosphate 4-kinase, type II, alpha (*PIP5K2A*) has been found to be involved in response to oxidative stress [93] and SCZ [20, 72]. A recent study on 491 patients from three clinical centres in Siberia has found an association between rs10828317, rs746203 and rs8341 variants of *PIP5K2A* to be protective variants against TD [21]. Further replications on independent samples are required to validate the association between *PIP5K2A* and TD.

2.2.1.4   Other Genes

Several replicated studies suggested an association between *BDNF*, *CNR1*, *DPP6* and *HSPG2* variants and TD, which are reviewed here.

The Brain-Derived Neurotrophic Factor (BDNF)

The *BDNF* gene codes for a neuronal growth peptide, involved in dopaminergic pathway and potentially in TD [96]. A recent meta-analysis has not confirmed numerous, previous associations between the *BDNF* Val66Met (rs6265) variant and TD [57]. Serum levels of BDNF have been found to be consistently decreased in TD patients [96]. Due to mixed results in genetic association studies and negative results from the most recent meta-analysis, the rs6265 is unlikely to play a major role in TD.

Cannabinoid Receptor 1 (CNR1)

Cannabinoid receptors have been implicated in movement disorders and are down-regulated in Huntington's disease, whereas upregulation is observed in Parkinson's disease [86]. Based on the mentioned observations, cannabinoid-based drugs targeting the cannabinoid-signalling systems are believed to alleviate motor symptoms [22] and make cannabinoid receptors ideal genes to be studied in the context of TD. A study by Tiwari et al. [86] has investigated the role of *CNR1* gene and TD;

initial report has shown association of the rs806374 in the *CNR1* gene and TD, with the CC genotype and C allele carriers to be more likely to develop TD. Additionally, these individuals have been also more likely to develop more severe clinical manifestations of TD [86]. This is the only study thus far to have investigated TD in relation to *CNR1*; further replications are required to validate this genetic association.

Dipeptidyl Peptidase-Like Protein 6 (DPP6)

DPP6 codes for a transmembrane protein that binds to voltage-gated potassium channels. Its protein may influence dopamine neurons. A recent GWAS discovered an association between *DPP6* variant rs6977820 and TD. This variant has been significantly linked to TD in both the discovery and replication samples [80]. The newly discovered gene variant rs6977820 decreased *DPP6* expression in the human postmortem prefrontal cortex [80], suggesting that low protein level of *DPP6* in the brain may be a risk factor for TD. This promising genetic association requires further replication studies, and cellular experiments are also encouraged to determine the molecular basis of this association in TD.

Heparan Sulphate Proteoglycan 2 (HSPG2), Perlecan

HSPG2 codes for a multidomain protein responsible for stabilisation of other molecules in the membrane, glomerular permeability to macromolecules, and cell adhesion. A GWAS from 2010 identified *HSPG2* to be nominally associated with TD in a small sample, with replication in a second sample. Additionally, the risk allele (rs2445142) was linked with higher expression of *HSPG2* in postmortem human prefrontal brain [79]. Initial findings have been later replicated in Caucasian Americans recruited as part of the CATIE study. Additionally, the G allele of rs2445142 has been found to be associated with TD in a Jewish-Israeli clinical cohort [26]. Initial results across the various studies have shown *HSPG2* rs2445142 as promising gene for the risk assessment of TD in the clinical setting. Further translational and clinical assessments are required before the *HSPG2* rs2445142 variant can become part of a genetic screening panel for TD (Table 2.1).

2.2.2   Antipsychotic-Induced Weight Gain (AIWG)

AIWG is a highly heritable ($h^2 = 0.6$–0.8) and polygenic side effect of atypical antipsychotics. AIWG risk differs amongst SGAPs with "high-risk" AIWG drugs including clozapine and olanzapine, "moderate risk" including risperidone and quetiapine, and haloperidol and aripiprazole being "low risk." Substantial weight gain leads to diabetes type II, metabolic syndrome, and cardiovascular diseases. AIWG

Table 2.1 Summary of most promising polymorphisms associated with tardive dyskinesia

Gene	Polymorphism	Main findings
CYP1A2	(*1F, −163C>A, rs762551)	CC genotype and/or C allele are possible risk factors for tardive dyskinesia
SLC18A2	rs2015586	C allele can be a risk variant for tardive dyskinesia
PIP5K2A	rs10828317	Association of CC genotype with tardive dyskinesia
CNR1	rs806374	Possible risk for tardive dyskinesia in C-allele carriers
DPP6	rs6977820	A allele was associated with tardive dyskinesia
HSPG2	rs2445142	G allele was associated with tardive dyskinesia

results in social stigmatisation of weight gain, leading to patient incompliance, which further increases the need to determine the aetiology to alleviate AIWG in AP-treated patients [50]. While there have been no significant AIWG findings with FGAP treatment due to lack of adequate samples thus far [18], several interesting findings were reported with SGAPs.

2.2.2.1 Neurotransmitter Genes

Some neurotransmitters (e.g. serotonin and dopamine) are highly involved in appetite regulation thus they have been predominantly chosen as good candidates for AIWG studies [76].

Serotonin System Genes

The serotonin system has been extensively analyzed in relation to AIWG, as serotonin receptors are one of the main targets of SGAPs [50]. Serotonin transporters also affect central pathways that influence satiety and hunger [50].

There are several consistent results that described an association between the functional HTR2C gene −759C/T (rs3813929) polymorphism and AIWG. Two meta-analyses have confirmed the role of −759C/T variant in AIWG [15, 54, 76]. The C allele has been suggested to be a risk variant as it has been found to be more frequent in AIWG cases than in control (non-AIWG) populations. However, the role of −759C/T in metabolic syndrome is less clear, as some studies have found associations with metabolic syndrome [28, 59], whereas other studies have failed to replicate the same findings [35, 70]. While a recent meta-analysis have not confirmed an association of −759C/T and metabolic syndrome, a strong trend has been shown for the C allele to be associated with high olanzapine-induced weight gain [54].

Several genetic association studies have been conducted with the intronic HTR2C variant rs1414334 and AIWG, albeit with mixed results. A positive link for rs1414334 has been established in a meta-analysis [54]; however, a recent study has not able to replicate the association between rs1414334 and AIWG [41].

Lack of replication may be due to the differences in the ethnicities of populations analyzed, medications prescribed, previous exposure to AP, and importantly length of treatment observation [94]. Thus, more studies with stringent sample selection are required to avoid confounding effects and increase likelihood of replicated findings.

Dopamine System Genes

The dopamine system plays an important role in mediating AP response; additionally, disruptions in *DRD2* have been linked with obesity [50].

The A allele of *DRD2* rs2440390 variant has shown association with more severe AIWG [30] in patients without SCZ; however, this finding awaits replication. A recent study on a Polish population showed no effect of the *DRD2* -141C Ins/Del (rs1799732), Taq1A, and *DRD2* exon 8 variants on AIWG during ziprasidone, olanzapine, and perazine treatment [91]. A previous study on first-episode patients treated with risperidone and olanzapine has shown the del allele to be associated with AIWG [48]. A later study has shown an association between three *DRD2* SNPs: rs6277 (or C957T), rs1079598 and rs1800497 (TaqIA), and AIWG [62]. Thus, some *DRD2* gene variants appear to be suggestive risk factors for AIWG. Gene-gene interaction or pathway analyses may help to validate these risk variants further and detect contribution of each variant.

2.2.2.2 Leptin and Leptin Receptor

Leptin is an adipocyte hormone that works as a long-term regulator of energy balance and is part of a negative feedback loop regulating body weight. Leptin released in adipose tissue signals the brain to decrease food intake and increase energy metabolism. Furthermore, mutations in the *LEP* gene have been reported in obesity and insulin resistance [7]. Taken together, leptin and its receptor are natural candidates for AIWG genetic studies.

The −2548A/G *LEP* gene variant has been reported to be associated with AIWG; however, studies produced inconsistent results. In a longitudinal (>1 year) study of an Asian population, the A allele and the AA genotype have been reported as risk factors for AIWG [34, 95]; however, other studies have suggested the G/A genotype to be the risk factor [34, 101]. In contrast, the G allele has been found to be associated with AIWG in a Caucasian sample [9, 19]. Further, replication studies have resulted in mostly negative results [7, 64]. A recent investigation on autistic children and adolescents treated with risperidone have shown increased AIWG risk for G allele carriers [63]. One recent meta-analysis study has yielded negative findings; however, studies were heterogeneous and phenotype definitions remained unclear [74]. Another recent retrospective association study in Finnish patients also yielded negative results [41]. Most plausible explanations for inconsistent findings are likely due to various ethnicities, different study durations, and heterogenous AP treatment. Significant associations have been mostly reported in Asian patients observed for longer time periods (>1 year), mostly on monotherapy. Although clinically significant weight gain may appear in the first weeks of treatment, study findings suggest at least 9 weeks of observation may be necessary to observe statistically significant genetic associations [81].

One study explored the gene-gene interaction between *LEP* (rs7799039) and leptin receptor, *LEPR* (Q223R) however, no significant interaction has been detected [7]. The Q223R *LEPR* variant was previously investigated in AIWG pharmacogenetic studies, albeit with mixed reuslts. The R allele and RR genotype have been associated with higher risk for obesity following AP treatment [19, 27]; however, other studies have failed to confirm the role of Q223R with AIWG [7, 67].

2.2.2.3 The Melanocortin 4 Receptor (MC4R)

The melanocortin 4 receptor (*MC4R*) gene locus has been shown to be one of the best and consistently replicated findings associated with AIWG [37, 73]. *MC4R* is a membrane-bound receptor that plays an essential role in the regulation of energy homeostasis [29]. Defects of *MC4R* are one of the causes for monogenic forms of obesity [29]. GWAS study of SGAP-treated sample has shown strong association of *MC4R* gene locus marker rs489693 in AIWG, which has been replicated in three independent samples [55]. In addition, the same variant has been associated with AIWG in another German study [13]. Notably, in a sample with children and adolescents treated with risperidone for autism symptoms, this marker has been again associated with AIWG, however, showing an opposite allele effect [63].

Other variants of the *MC4R* gene have been investigated in AIWG, including *MC4R* variant rs8087522. The A-allele carriers gained more weight than noncarriers. Results became marginal after correction for multiple testing; however, in vitro studies have suggested that the A allele might create a binding site for transcription factors [12].

2.2.2.4 The Cannabinoid Receptor 1 (*CNR1*) and the Neuropeptide Y (*NPY*) Genes

The cannabinoid receptor 1 (*CNR1*) is associated with appetite and satiety. One study has showed an association between *CNR1* rs806378 variant and AIWG, in which T-allele carriers have been found to gain more weight than CC carriers [85]. Notably, another study in autism children and adolescents has shown the same trend for the T allele [63].

Based on the association with *CNR1*, Tiwari et al. conducted a study investigating the neuropeptide Y (*NPY*) gene since it has shown to interact with *CNR1* in animal studies [82]. *NPY* is an orexigenic peptide that stimulates food intake [82]. This study has found an interaction with *NPY* rs16147 and *CNR1* rs806378 to be associated with AIWG [82].

2.2.2.5 Mitochondrial Genes

The mitochondria plays a key role in energy homeostasis, and it has been shown to be related with neuronal activity [36] and obesity [42]. Recently the rs6971 variant of the translocator protein 18kDA *(TSPO)* has been found to be associated with AIWG in two independent samples [68]. In another study, associations have been found between rs6435326 variant of NADH dehydrogenase (ubiquinone) Fe-S protein 1 *(NDUFS1)* and AIWG in two independent samples [25]. Furthermore, this study also discovered a significant gene-gene interaction between the TT genotype of rs6435326 and the AG genotype of rs3762883 of the cytochrome C oxidase assembly factor *(COX18)* [25]. These are the first studies conducted with mitochondrial genes to suggest that they may have a significant role in AIWG.

2.2.2.6 Other Genes

Few studies have investigated associations between other genes and AIWG. One such gene is the *BDNF* gene in relation to AIWG. The Val/Val (rs6265) genotype of *BDNF* has been found to be associated with increased AIWG in Han Chinese, risperidone-treated sample [45]. However, a study on a larger Asian sample has failed to replicate the original findings [87] but has reported an association of AIWG with another *BDNF* variant rs11030101. Subsequent analysis has shown association of *BDNF* haplotype rs6265-rs1519480 with strong, nominal association between Val/Val genotype and AIWG [100]. In summary, *BDNF* gene variants might be associated with AIWG; however, the genetic architecture of the *BDNF* gene requires further investigation.

The methylenetetrahydrofolate reductase *(MTHFR)* is involved in the homocysteine metabolism and thus potentially associated with AIWG [78]. The CC genotype of 677C/T (rs1801133) variant has been linked to significant AP-induced increase in BMI in both Spanish and Chinese samples [78]. An independent study has confirmed a possible risk of the C allele in both chronic and first-episode patients [38].

In 2011, a GWAS study of 738 patients, investigating 492 000 SNPs, has found an association between meis homeobox 2 *(MEIS2)*, cyclic adenosine monophosphate-dependent, regulatory, type II, beta *(PRKAR2B)*, forming homology 2 domain containing 3 *(FHOD3)*, ring finger protein 144A *(RNF144A, ASTN2)*, sex-determining region Y-box 5 *(SOX5)*, and activating transcription factor 7 interacting protein 2 *(ATF7IP2)* and AIWG [1]. However, replication studies for the mentioned genes are still need to be conducted for validation.

Our group recently submitted a GWAS study conducted on a well-characterised, genetically homogenous subsample of European ancestry carefully selected from CATIE study. None of the variants from this study have reached genome-wide significance; however, strong, nominal associations were found for rs9346455 located upstream of opioid growth factor receptor-like 1 *(OGFRL1)* and rs1059778 located in iron-sulfur cluster assembly *(IBA57)*. In addition, we investigated our top hit findings in a smaller replication cohort, in which the top SNP rs9346455 has shown

Table 2.2 Summary of most promising polymorphisms associated with antipsychotic-induced weight gain

Gene	Polymorphism	Main findings
HTR2C	−759C/T (rs3813929)	The C allele was suggested to be a risk variant
LEP	−2548A/G	The A allele is a risk factor for antipsychotic-induced weight gain in Asians, whereas G allele is linked to antipsychotic-induced weight gain in Caucasians. Results were significant only in longitudinal studies of extended duration
MC4R	rs489693	AA genotype associated with increased weight gain
CNR1	rs806378	T allele associated with antipsychotic-induced weight gain
NDUFS1	rs1801318	TT genotype associated with increased weight gain

significant association with AIWG. The combined meta-analysis p-value for rs9346455 was close to genome-wide significance ($p < 10^{-7}$) [8a] (Table 2.2).

2.2.3   Clozapine-Induced Agranulocytosis (CIA)

Clozapine-induced agranulocytosis (CIA) is a severe adverse effect in treatment-resistant SCZ patient population requiring clozapine. CIA is present in up to 2 % of clozapine-treated SCZ patients [8]. It is usually linked with the immune-mediated response against neutrophils and toxic effect against bone marrow stromal cells [8].

Most studies have linked CIA to the human leucocyte antigen (HLA) system genes, which are part of the major histocompatibility complex (MHC). HLA genes have been linked with several immune and nonimmune diseases, and adverse drug reactions to xenobiotics [90]. The strongest CIA associations exist for HLA-DQB1 and HLA-B38 variants; however, the effects of particular genes and genetic variants in CIA are poorly replicated [8, 11]. The myeloperoxidase (MPO) and nicotinamide adenine dinucleotide phosphate oxidase (NOX) have also been suggested to be associated with CIA, albeit results are not as consistent as for HLA [8]. Meanwhile, another recent paper published on CIA in a Finnish sample using whole-exome sequencing identified protein tyrosine phosphatase, receptor type, f polypeptide, interacting protein, alpha 4 (PPFIA4), ubiquitin specific peptidase 43 (USP43), actinin, alpha 1 (ACTN1), podocan-like 1 (PODNL1), and spermatogenesis associated, serine-rich 1 (SPATS1) as the top five hits [84]. Although these genes have not reached whole-exome significance, they show a trend towards immunologically associated genes in CIA.

One GWAS has suggested a role of MyoD family inhibitor domain containing (MDFIC) and proteoglycan 4 (PRG4) loci in risk for CIA [16]. Further replications are required to validate these results.

Of note, in 2007, a first commercial test kit for CIA, the PGxPredict:CLOZAPINE test (Clinical Data, Inc, New Haven, CT) was launched. The test reached a high specificity of 98.4 % but sensitivity scores remained low at 21.5 %, thus failing to detect patients at high risk for CIA [8]. More pharmacogenetic research is needed to develop newer and more precise genetic screening tests for patients. Polygenic risk scores, derived from gene-gene interaction studies, may improve the initial algorithm.

2.3 Summary

Genetic associations of common and serious AP side effects have been extensively studied in the recent years. As for TD, gene variants in *CYP1A2*, *SLC18A2¹PIP5K2A*, *CNR1, DPP6,* and *HSPG2* have yielded promising results. However, this area of research would substantially benefit from further investigation in larger, well-characterised samples allowing for additional GWAS.

For AIWG, *HTR2C*, *LEP*, *MC4R*, *NDUFS1*, and *CNR1* have recently yielded the strongest findings. The most clinically relevant finding was obtained in *MC4R* homozygote carriers for rs489693 who on average gained twice as much weight than noncarriers. In addition to other risk variants, such as *HTR2C*, polygenic risk tests for AIWG might become available for use in clinical practice.

As for CIA, a few studies have been conducted in the past years linking CIA further to immunological system genes. These findings suggest that gene variants associated with CIA might show relatively large effect sizes such as the *HLA-B*15:02* allele which is associated with an increased risk of carbamazepine-induced Stevens-Johnson syndrome [46]. While an early genetic test for CIA failed to detect high-risk group due to low sensitivity, it is very likely that further research will aid in developing an improved genetic test to predict patients at risk for CIA. This would allow for the discontinuation of regular blood draws required to screen for the development of CIA.

In reviewing the literature, certain limitations in these genetic studies need to be addressed. The samples used were relatively small compared to disease genetic studies since high-standard pharmacogenetic studies require the collection of prospectively assessed samples. However, in many cases, genes involved in response and side effects to medication often show larger effect sizes than disease-risk genes. Many genetic association analyses faced issues with heterogeneity, either caused by ancestry and/or by current/previous medication exposure. Given these limitations, it is important to conduct more studies with standardised methodologies to obtain more consistent and comparable results, to develop new or refine existing genetic tests. First tests have been introduced mainly to identify nonnormal metabolizers for CYP enzymes (particularly for *CYP2D6*) to optimise AP drug treatment. The United States Food and Drug Administration (FDA) labelled over 100 medications for genetic testing, including 32 in psychiatry/neurology [17]. Expert groups such as the Clinical Pharmacogenetics Implementation Consortium (CPIC) are providing guidelines to help clinicians use genetic information to select type/dosage of various drugs to decrease trial-and-error switches in medications [10].

Future studies should analyse gene-gene interactions in order to explain higher degree of variants. More studies with stringent sample selection are required to avoid confounding effects (e.g. assessing medication exposure, considering ethnic differences) in order to increase the likelihood to replicate initial findings. Nonetheless, research in pharmacogenetics of APs have made some substantial progresses in the past years raising hope for an accelerated development of genetic testing in clinical practice.

References

1. Adkins DE, Aberg K, McClay JL, Bukszar J, Zhao Z, Jia P et al (2011) Genomewide pharmacogenomic study of metabolic side effects to antipsychotic drugs. Mol Psychiatry 16(3):321–332
2. Al Hadithy AF, Ivanova SA, Pechlivanoglou P, Semke A, Fedorenko O et al (2009) Tardive dyskinesia and DRD3, HTR2A and HTR2C gene polymorphisms in Russian psychiatric inpatients from Siberia. Prog Neuropsychopharmacol Biol Psychiatry 33(3):475–481
3. Bakker PR, Al Hadithy AF, Amin N, van Duijn CM, van Os J, van Harten PN (2012) Antipsychotic-induced movement disorders in long-stay psychiatric patients and 45 tag SNPs in 7 candidate genes: a prospective study. PLoS One 7(12):e50970
4. Bakker PR, van Harten PN, van Os J (2008) Antipsychotic-induced tardive dyskinesia and polymorphic variations in COMT, DRD2, CYP1A2 and MnSOD genes: a meta-analysis of pharmacogenetic interactions. Mol Psychiatry 13(5):544–556
5. Basile VS, Masellis M, Potkin SG, Kennedy JL (2002) Pharmacogenomics in schizophrenia: the quest for individualized therapy. Hum Mol Genet 11(20):2517–2530
6. Boskovic M, Vovk T, Saje M, Goricar K, Dolzan V, Kores Plesnicar B, Grabnar I (2013) Association of SOD2, GPX1, CAT, and TNF genetic polymorphisms with oxidative stress, neurochemistry, psychopathology, and extrapyramidal symptoms in schizophrenia. Neurochem Res 38(2):433–442
7. Brandl EJ, Frydrychowicz C, Tiwari AK, Lett TA, Kitzrow W, Buttner S et al (2012) Association study of polymorphisms in leptin and leptin receptor genes with antipsychotic-induced body weight gain. Prog Neuropsychopharmacol Biol Psychiatry 38(2):134–141
8. Brandl EJ, Kennedy JL, Muller DJ (2014) Pharmacogenetics of antipsychotics. Can J Psychiatry 59(2):76–88
8a. Brandl EJ, Tiwari AK, Zai CC, Nurmi EL, Chowdhury NI, Arenovich T, Sanches M, Goncalves VF, Shen JJ, Lieberman JA, Meltzer HY, Kennedy JL, Müller DJ. Genome-wide association study on antipsychotic-induced weight gain in the CATIE sample. Pharmacogenomics J (in press)
9. Calarge CA, Ellingrod VL, Zimmerman B, Acion L, Sivitz WI, Schlechte JA (2009) Leptin gene -2548G/A variants predict risperidone-associated weight gain in children and adolescents. Psychiatr Genet 19(6):320–327
10. Caudle KE, Klein TE, Hoffman JM, Muller DJ, Whirl-Carrillo M, Gong L et al (2014) Incorporation of pharmacogenomics into routine clinical practice: the Clinical Pharmacogenetics Implementation Consortium (CPIC) guideline development process. Curr Drug Metab 15(2):209–217
11. Chowdhury NI, Remington G, Kennedy JL (2011) Genetics of antipsychotic-induced side effects and agranulocytosis. Curr Psychiatry Rep 13(2):156–165
12. Chowdhury NI, Tiwari AK, Souza RP, Zai CC, Shaikh SA, Chen S et al (2013) Genetic association study between antipsychotic-induced weight gain and the melanocortin-4 receptor gene. Pharmacogenomics J 13(3):272–279
13. Czerwensky F, Leucht S, Steimer W (2013) Association of the common MC4R rs17782313 polymorphism with antipsychotic-related weight gain. J Clin Psychopharmacol 33(1): 74–79

14. de Leon J, Susce MT, Pan RM, Koch WH, Wedlund PJ (2005) Polymorphic variations in GSTM1, GSTT1, PgP, CYP2D6, CYP3A5, and dopamine D2 and D3 receptors and their association with tardive dyskinesia in severe mental illness. J Clin Psychopharmacol 25(5):448–456

15. De Luca V, Mueller DJ, de Bartolomeis A, Kennedy JL (2007) Association of the HTR2C gene and antipsychotic induced weight gain: a meta-analysis. Int J Neuropsychopharmacol 10(5):697–704

16. de With SA, Pulit SL, Wang T, Staal WG, van Solinge WW, de Bakker PI, Ophoff RA (2015) Genome-wide association study of lymphoblast cell viability after clozapine exposure. Am J Med Genet B Neuropsychiatr Genet 168(2):116–122

17. Drozda K, Muller DJ, Bishop JR (2014) Pharmacogenomic testing for neuropsychiatric drugs: current status of drug labeling, guidelines for using genetic information, and test options. Pharmacotherapy 34(2):166–184

18. Ebert T, Midbari Y, Shmilovitz R, Kosov I, Kotler M, Weizman A, Ram A (2014) Metabolic effects of antipsychotics in prepubertal children: a retrospective chart review. J Child Adolesc Psychopharmacol 24(4):218–222

19. Ellingrod VL, Bishop JR, Moline J, Lin YC, Miller DD (2007) Leptin and leptin receptor gene polymorphisms and increases in body mass index (BMI) from olanzapine treatment in persons with schizophrenia. Psychopharmacol Bull 40(1):57–62

20. Fedorenko O, Rudikov EV, Gavrilova VA, Boiarko EG, Semke AV, Ivanova SA (2013) Association of (N251S)-PIP5K2A with schizophrenic disorders: a study of the Russian population of Siberia. Zh Nevrol Psikhiatr Im S S Korsakova 113(5):58–61

21. Fedorenko OY, Loonen AJ, Lang F, Toshchakova VA, Boyarko EG, Semke AV, et al. (2015) Association study indicates a protective role of phosphatidylinositol-4-phosphate-5-kinase against tardive dyskinesia. Int J Neuropsychopharmacol 18(6):1–6

22. Fernandez-Ruiz J (2009) The endocannabinoid system as a target for the treatment of motor dysfunction. Br J Pharmacol 156(7):1029–1040

23. Fu Y, Fan CH, Deng HH, Hu SH, Lv DP, Li LH et al (2006) Association of CYP2D6 and CYP1A2 gene polymorphism with tardive dyskinesia in Chinese schizophrenic patients. Acta Pharmacol Sin 27(3):328–332

24. Gaedigk A (2013) Complexities of CYP2D6 gene analysis and interpretation. Int Rev Psychiatry 25(5):534–553

25. Goncalves VF, Zai CC, Tiwari AK, Brandl EJ, Derkach A, Meltzer HY et al (2014) A hypothesis-driven association study of 28 nuclear-encoded mitochondrial genes with antipsychotic-induced weight gain in schizophrenia. Neuropsychopharmacology 39(6):1347–1354

26. Greenbaum L, Alkelai A, Zozulinsky P, Kohn Y, Lerer B (2012) Support for association of HSPG2 with tardive dyskinesia in Caucasian populations. Pharmacogenomics J 12(6):513–520

27. Gregoor JG, van der Weide J, Loovers HM, van Megen HJ, Egberts TC, Heerdink ER (2011) Polymorphisms of the LEP, LEPR and HTR2C gene: obesity and BMI change in patients using antipsychotic medication in a naturalistic setting. Pharmacogenomics 12(6):919–923

28. Gunes A, Melkersson KI, Scordo MG, Dahl ML (2009) Association between HTR2C and HTR2A polymorphisms and metabolic abnormalities in patients treated with olanzapine or clozapine. J Clin Psychopharmacol 29(1):65–68

29. He S, Tao YX (2014) Defect in MAPK signaling as a cause for monogenic obesity caused by inactivating mutations in the melanocortin-4 receptor gene. Int J Biol Sci 10(10):1128–1137

30. Houston JP, Kohler J, Bishop JR, Ellingrod VL, Ostbye KM, Zhao F et al (2012) Pharmacogenomic associations with weight gain in olanzapine treatment of patients without schizophrenia. J Clin Psychiatry 73(8):1077–1086

31. Hsieh CJ, Chen YC, Lai MS, Hong CJ, Chien KL (2011) Genetic variability in serotonin receptor and transporter genes may influence risk for tardive dyskinesia in chronic schizophrenia. Psychiatry Res 188(1):175–176

32. Ivanova SA, Toshchakova VA, Filipenko ML, Fedorenko OY, Boyarko EG, Boiko AS et al (2015) Cytochrome P450 1A2 co-determines neuroleptic load and may diminish tardive dyskinesia by increased inducibility. World J Biol Psychiatry 16(3):200–205

33. Janno S, Holi M, Tuisku K, Wahlbeck K (2004) Prevalence of neuroleptic-induced movement disorders in chronic schizophrenia inpatients. Am J Psychiatry 161(1):160–163

34. Kang SG, Lee HJ, Park YM, Choi JE, Han C, Kim YK et al (2008) Possible association between the -2548A/G polymorphism of the leptin gene and olanzapine-induced weight gain. Prog Neuropsychopharmacol Biol Psychiatry 32(1):160–163

35. Kang SH, Lee JI, Chang AK, Joo YH, Kim CY, Kim SY (2011) Genetic polymorphisms in the HTR2C and peroxisome proliferator-activated receptors are not associated with metabolic syndrome in patients with schizophrenia taking Clozapine. Psychiatry Investig 8(3):262–268

36. Kann O, Kovacs R (2007) Mitochondria and neuronal activity. Am J Physiol Cell Physiol 292(2):C641–C657

37. Kao AC, Muller DJ (2013) Genetics of antipsychotic-induced weight gain: update and current perspectives. Pharmacogenomics 14(16):2067–2083

38. Kao AC, Rojnic Kuzman M, Tiwari AK, Zivkovic MV, Chowdhury NI, Medved V et al (2014) Methylenetetrahydrofolate reductase gene variants and antipsychotic-induced weight gain and metabolic disturbances. J Psychiatr Res 54:36–42

39. Kapur S, Seeman P (2001) Does fast dissociation from the dopamine D(2) receptor explain the action of atypical antipsychotics?: a new hypothesis. Am J Psychiatry 158(3):360–369

40. Kapur S, Zipursky R, Jones C, Remington G, Houle S (2000) Relationship between dopamine D(2) occupancy, clinical response, and side effects: a double-blind PET study of first-episode schizophrenia. Am J Psychiatry 157(4):514–520

41. Klemettila JP, Kampman O, Seppala N, Viikki M, Hamalainen M, Moilanen E et al (2015) Association study of the HTR2C, leptin and adiponectin genes and serum marker analyses in clozapine treated long-term patients with schizophrenia. Eur Psychiatry 30(2):296–302

42. Knoll N, Jarick I, Volckmar AL, Klingenspor M, Illig T, Grallert H et al (2014) Mitochondrial DNA variants in obesity. PLoS One 9(5):e94882

43. Koning JP, Vehof J, Burger H, Wilffert B, Al Hadithy A, Alizadeh B et al (2012) Association of two DRD2 gene polymorphisms with acute and tardive antipsychotic-induced movement disorders in young Caucasian patients. Psychopharmacology (Berl) 219(3):727–736

44. Koola MM, Tsapakis EM, Wright P, Smith S, Kerwin Rip RW, Nugent KL, Aitchison KJ (2014) Association of tardive dyskinesia with variation in CYP2D6: is there a role for active metabolites? J Psychopharmacol 28(7):665–670

45. Lane HY, Liu YC, Huang CL, Chang YC, Wu PL, Lu CT, Chang WH (2006) Risperidone-related weight gain: genetic and nongenetic predictors. J Clin Psychopharmacol 26(2):128–134

46. Leckband SG, Kelsoe JR, Dunnenberger HM, George AL Jr, Tran E, Berger R, Muller DJ et al (2013) Clinical pharmacogenetics implementation consortium guidelines for HLA-B genotype and carbamazepine dosing. Clin Pharmacol Ther 94(3):324–328

47. Lee HJ, Kang SG (2011) Genetics of tardive dyskinesia. Int Rev Neurobiol 98:231–264

48. Lencz T, Robinson DG, Napolitano B, Sevy S, Kane JM, Goldman D, Malhotra AK (2010) DRD2 promoter region variation predicts antipsychotic-induced weight gain in first episode schizophrenia. Pharmacogenet Genomics 20(9):569–572

49. Lerer B, Segman RH, Tan EC, Basile VS, Cavallaro R, Aschauer HN et al (2005) Combined analysis of 635 patients confirms an age-related association of the serotonin 2A receptor gene with tardive dyskinesia and specificity for the non-orofacial subtype. Int J Neuropsychopharmacol 8(3):411–425

50. Lett TA, Wallace TJ, Chowdhury NI, Tiwari AK, Kennedy JL, Muller DJ (2012) Pharmacogenetics of antipsychotic-induced weight gain: review and clinical implications. Mol Psychiatry 17(3):242–266

51. Liou YJ, Liao DL, Chen JY, Wang YC, Lin CC, Bai YM, Yu SC, Lin MW, Lai IC (2004) Association analysis of the dopamine D3 receptor gene ser9gly and brain-derived neurotrophic

factor gene val66met polymorphisms with antipsychotic-induced persistent tardive dyskinesia and clinical expression in Chinese schizophrenic patients. Neuromolecular Med 5(3):243–251

52. Liu H, Wang C, Chen PH, Zhang BS, Zheng YL, Zhang CX et al (2010) Association of the manganese superoxide dismutase gene Ala-9Val polymorphism with clinical phenotypes and tardive dyskinesia in schizophrenic patients. Prog Neuropsychopharmacol Biol Psychiatry 34(4):692–696

53. Lohmann PL, Bagli M, Krauss H, Muller DJ, Schulze TG, Fangerau H et al (2003) CYP2D6 polymorphism and tardive dyskinesia in schizophrenic patients. Pharmacopsychiatry 36(2): 73–78

54. Ma X, Maimaitirexiati T, Zhang R, Gui X, Zhang W, Xu G, Hu G (2014) HTR2C polymorphisms, olanzapine-induced weight gain and antipsychotic-induced metabolic syndrome in schizophrenia patients: a meta-analysis. Int J Psychiatry Clin Pract 18(4):229–242

55. Malhotra AK, Correll CU, Chowdhury NI, Muller DJ, Gregersen PK, Lee AT et al (2012) Association between common variants near the melanocortin 4 receptor gene and severe antipsychotic drug-induced weight gain. Arch Gen Psychiatry 69(9):904–912

56. Meltzer HY (1999) The role of serotonin in antipsychotic drug action. Neuropsychopharmacology 21(2 Suppl):106S–115S

57. Miura I, Zhang JP, Nitta M, Lencz T, Kane JM, Malhotra AK, Yabe H, Correll CU (2014) BDNF Val66Met polymorphism and antipsychotic-induced tardive dyskinesia occurrence and severity: a meta-analysis. Schizophr Res 152(2–3):365–372

58. Miyamoto S, Duncan GE, Marx CE, Lieberman JA (2005) Treatments for schizophrenia: a critical review of pharmacology and mechanisms of action of antipsychotic drugs. Mol Psychiatry 10(1):79–104

59. Mulder H, Franke B, van der-Beek van der AA, Arends J, Wilmink FW, Egberts AC, Scheffer H (2007) The association between HTR2C polymorphisms and obesity in psychiatric patients using antipsychotics: a cross-sectional study. Pharmacogenomics J 5:318–324

60. Muller DJ, Kekin I, Kao AC, Brandl EJ (2013) Towards the implementation of CYP2D6 and CYP2C19 genotypes in clinical practice: update and report from a pharmacogenetic service clinic. Int Rev Psychiatry 25(5):554–571

61. Muller DJ, Schulze TG, Knapp M, Held T, Krauss H, Weber T et al (2001) Familial occurrence of tardive dyskinesia. Acta Psychiatr Scand 104(5):375–379

62. Muller DJ, Zai CC, Sicard M, Remington E, Souza RP, Tiwari AK et al (2012) Systematic analysis of dopamine receptor genes (DRD1-DRD5) in antipsychotic-induced weight gain. Pharmacogenomics J 12(2):156–164

63. Nurmi EL, Spilman SL, Whelan F, Scahill LL, Aman MG, McDougle CJ et al (2013) Moderation of antipsychotic-induced weight gain by energy balance gene variants in the RUPP autism network risperidone studies. Transl Psychiatry 3:e274

64. Opgen-Rhein C, Brandl EJ, Muller DJ, Neuhaus AH, Tiwari AK, Sander T, Dettling M (2010) Association of HTR2C, but not LEP or INSIG2, genes with antipsychotic-induced weight gain in a German sample. Pharmacogenomics 11(6):773–780

65. Park YM, Kang SG, Choi JE, Kim YK, Kim SH, Park JY, Kim L, Lee HJ (2011) No evidence for an association between Dopamine D2 receptor polymorphisms and Tardive Dyskinesia in Korean Schizophrenia patients. Psychiatry Investig 8(1):49–54

66. Patsopoulos NA, Ntzani EE, Zintzaras E, Ioannidis JP (2005) CYP2D6 polymorphisms and the risk of tardive dyskinesia in schizophrenia: a meta-analysis. Pharmacogenet Genomics 15(3):151–158

67. Perez-Iglesias R, Mata I, Amado JA, Berja A, Garcia-Unzueta MT, Martinez Garcia O et al (2010) Effect of FTO, SH2B1, LEP, and LEPR polymorphisms on weight gain associated with antipsychotic treatment. J Clin Psychopharmacol 30(6):661–666

68. Pouget JG, Goncalves VF, Nurmi EL, P.Laughlin C, Mallya KS, McCracken JT et al (2015) Investigation of TSPO variants in schizophrenia and antipsychotic treatment outcomes. Pharmacogenomics 16(1):5–22

69. Renou J, De Luca V, Zai CC, Bulgin N, Remington G, Meltzer HY, Lieberman JA, Le Foll B, Kennedy JL (2007) Multiple variants of the DRD3, but not BDNF gene, influence age-at-onset of schizophrenia. Mol Psychiatry 12(12):1058–1060

70. Risselada AJ, Vehof J, Bruggeman R, Wilffert B, Cohen D, Al Hadithy AF, Arends J, Mulder H (2012) Association between HTR2C gene polymorphisms and the metabolic syndrome in patients using antipsychotics: a replication study. Pharmacogenomics J 12(1):62–67

71. Rizos EN, Siafakas N, Katsantoni E, Lazou V, Sakellaropoulos K, Kastania A et al (2009) Association of the dopamine D3 receptor Ser9Gly and of the serotonin 2C receptor gene polymorphisms with tardive dyskinesia in Greeks with chronic schizophrenic disorder. Psychiatr Genet 19(2):106–107

72. Schwab SG, Knapp M, Sklar P, Eckstein GN, Sewekow C, Borrmann-Hassenbach M et al (2006) Evidence for association of DNA sequence variants in the phosphatidylinositol-4-phosphate 5-kinase IIalpha gene (PIP5K2A) with schizophrenia. Mol Psychiatry 11(9): 837–846

73. Shams TA, Muller DJ (2014) Antipsychotic induced weight gain: genetics, epigenetics, and biomarkers reviewed. Curr Psychiatry Rep 16(10):473

74. Shen J, Ge W, Zhang J, Zhu HJ, Fang Y (2014) Leptin -2548g/a gene polymorphism in association with antipsychotic-induced weight gain: a meta-analysis study. Psychiatr Danub 26(2):145–151

75. Shuman MD, Trigoboff E, Demler TL, Opler LA (2014) Exploring the potential effect of polypharmacy on the hematologic profiles of clozapine patients. J Psychiatr Pract 20(1): 50–58. doi:10.1097/01.pra.0000442937.61575.26

76. Sicard MN, Zai CC, Tiwari AK, Souza RP, Meltzer HY, Lieberman JA, Kennedy JL, Muller DJ (2010) Polymorphisms of the HTR2C gene and antipsychotic-induced weight gain: an update and meta-analysis. Pharmacogenomics 11(11):1561–1571. doi:10.2217/pgs.10.123

77. Soares-Weiser K, Fernandez HH (2007) Tardive dyskinesia. Semin Neurol 27(2):159–169. doi:10.1055/s-2007-971169

78. Srisawat U, Reynolds GP, Zhang ZJ, Zhang XR, Arranz B, San L, Dalton CF (2014) Methylenetetrahydrofolate reductase (MTHFR) 677C/T polymorphism is associated with antipsychotic-induced weight gain in first-episode schizophrenia. Int J Neuropsychopharmacol 17(3):485–490

79. Syu A, Ishiguro H, Inada T, Horiuchi Y, Tanaka S, Ishikawa M et al (2010) Association of the HSPG2 gene with neuroleptic-induced tardive dyskinesia. Neuropsychopharmacology 35(5):1155–1164

80. Tanaka S, Syu A, Ishiguro H, Inada T, Horiuchi Y, Ishikawa M et al (2013) DPP6 as a candidate gene for neuroleptic-induced tardive dyskinesia. Pharmacogenomics J 13(1):27–34

81. Templeman LA, Reynolds GP, Arranz B, San L (2005) Polymorphisms of the 5-HT2C receptor and leptin genes are associated with antipsychotic drug-induced weight gain in Caucasian subjects with a first-episode psychosis. Pharmacogenet Genomics 15(4):1 95–200

82. Tiwari AK, Brandl EJ, Weber C, Likhodi O, Zai CC, Hahn MK, Lieberman JA, Meltzer HY, Kennedy JL, Muller DJ (2013) Association of a functional polymorphism in neuropeptide Y with antipsychotic-induced weight gain in schizophrenia patients. J Clin Psychopharmacol 33(1):11–17

83. Tiwari AK, Deshpande SN, Rao AR, Bhatia T, Mukit SR, Shriharsh V, Lerer B, Nimagaonkar VL, Thelma BK (2005) Genetic susceptibility to tardive dyskinesia in chronic schizophrenia subjects: I. Association of CYP1A2 gene polymorphism. Pharmacogenomics J 5(1):60–69

84. Tiwari AK, Need AC, Lohoff FW, Zai CC, Chowdhury NI, Muller DJ et al (2014) Exome sequence analysis of Finnish patients with clozapine-induced agranulocytosis. Mol Psychiatry 19(4):403–405

85. Tiwari AK, Zai CC, Likhodi O, Lisker A, Singh D, Souza RP et al (2010) A common polymorphism in the cannabinoid receptor 1 (CNR1) gene is associated with antipsychotic-induced weight gain in Schizophrenia. Neuropsychopharmacology 35(6):1315–1324

86. Tiwari AK, Zai CC, Likhodi O, Voineskos AN, Meltzer HY, Lieberman JA et al (2012) Association study of cannabinoid receptor 1 (CNR1) gene in tardive dyskinesia. Pharmacogenomics J 12(3):260–266

87. Tsai A, Liou YJ, Hong CJ, Wu CL, Tsai SJ, Bai YM (2011) Association study of brain-derived neurotrophic factor gene polymorphisms and body weight change in schizophrenic patients under long-term atypical antipsychotic treatment. Neuromolecular Med 13(4): 328–333

88. Tsai HT, Caroff SN, Miller DD, McEvoy J, Lieberman JA, North KE, Stroup TS, Sullivan PF (2010) A candidate gene study of Tardive dyskinesia in the CATIE schizophrenia trial. Am J Med Genet B Neuropsychiatr Genet 153B(1):336–340

89. Tsai HT, North KE, West SL, Poole C (2010) The DRD3 rs6280 polymorphism and prevalence of tardive dyskinesia: a meta-analysis. Am J Med Genet B Neuropsychiatr Genet 153B(1):57–66

90. Turbay D, Lieberman J, Alper CA, Delgado JC, Corzo D, Yunis JJ, Yunis EJ (1997) Tumor necrosis factor constellation polymorphism and clozapine-induced agranulocytosis in two different ethnic groups. Blood 89(11):4167–4174

91. Tybura P, Trzesniowska-Drukala B, Bienkowski P, Beszlej A, Frydecka D, Mierzejewski P et al (2014) Pharmacogenetics of adverse events in schizophrenia treatment: comparison study of ziprasidone, olanzapine and perazine. Psychiatry Res 219(2):261–267

92. Utsuńomiya K, Shinkai T, Sakata S, Yamada K, Chen HI, De Luca V, Hwang R, Ohmori O, Nakamura J (2012) Genetic association between the dopamine D3 receptor gene polymorphism (Ser9Gly) and tardive dyskinesia in patients with schizophrenia: a reevaluation in East Asian populations. Neurosci Lett 507(1):52–56

93. van den Bout I, Divecha N (2009) PIP5K-driven PtdIns(4,5)P2 synthesis: regulation and cellular functions. J Cell Sci 122(Pt 21):3837–3850

94. Wallace TJ, Zai CC, Brandl EJ, Muller DJ (2011) Role of 5-HT(2C) receptor gene variants in antipsychotic-induced weight gain. Pharmgenomics Pers Med 4:83–93

95. Wu R, Zhao J, Shao P, Ou J, Chang M (2011) Genetic predictors of antipsychotic-induced weight gain: a case-matched multi-gene study. Zhong Nan Da Xue Xue Bao Yi Xue Ban 36(8):720–723

96. Yang YQ, Sun S, Yu YQ, Li WJ, Zhang X, Xiu MH et al (2011) Decreased serum brain-derived neurotrophic factor levels in schizophrenic patients with tardive dyskinesia. Neurosci Lett 502(1):37–40

97. Zai CC, De Luca V, Hwang RW, Voineskos A, Muller DJ, Remington G, Kennedy JL (2007) Meta-analysis of two dopamine D2 receptor gene polymorphisms with tardive dyskinesia in schizophrenia patients. Mol Psychiatry 12(9):794–795

98. Zai CC, Tiwari AK, Basile V, de Luca V, Muller DJ, Voineskos AN et al (2010) Oxidative stress in tardive dyskinesia: genetic association study and meta-analysis of NADPH quinine oxidoreductase 1 (NQO1) and Superoxide dismutase 2 (SOD2, MnSOD) genes. Prog Neuropsychopharmacol Biol Psychiatry 34(1):50–56

99. Zai CC, Tiwari AK, Mazzoco M, de Luca V, Muller DJ, Shaikh SA et al (2013) Association study of the vesicular monoamine transporter gene SLC18A2 with tardive dyskinesia. J Psychiatr Res 47(11):1760–1765

100. Zai GC, Zai CC, Chowdhury NI, Tiwari AK, Souza RP, Lieberman JA et al (2012) The role of brain-derived neurotrophic factor (BDNF) gene variants in antipsychotic response and antipsychotic-induced weight gain. Prog Neuropsychopharmacol Biol Psychiatry 39(1): 96–101

101. Zhang XY, Tan YL, Zhou DF, Haile CN, Cao LY, Xu Q, Shen Y, Kosten TA, Kosten TR (2007) Association of clozapine-induced weight gain with a polymorphism in the leptin promoter region in patients with chronic schizophrenia in a Chinese population. J Clin Psychopharmacol 27(3):246–251

Chapter 3
Pharmacogenetics of the Efficacy and Side Effects of Antidepressant Drugs

Chiara Fabbri and Alessandro Serretti

Abstract Both major depressive disorder (MDD) and antidepressant drug efficacy show an established evidence of being significantly affected by genetic polymorphisms. Thus, the pharmacogenetics of antidepressants has developed since the 1990s as a promising tool to produce tailored treatments of MDD.

Candidate gene studies were focused on a limited number of genes that were suggested to be involved in antidepressant mechanisms of action by preclinical evidence. Particularly, candidate studies provided quite replicated findings for the serotonin transporter gene (SLC6A4), brain-derived neurotrophic factor (BDNF), some subtypes of serotonin receptors (e.g., HTR2A), and genes involved in antidepressant metabolism and transport (e.g., ABCB1). Genome-wide association studies (GWAS) overcame the need of any a priori hypothesis and allowed the study of hundreds of thousands of polymorphisms throughout the whole genome. GWAS provided interesting signals in some individual genes (e.g., IL-11, NRG1, and RORA), but they also allowed to carry out more comprehensive analysis (e.g., pathway analysis), opening new perspectives.

Some pilot studies recently supported the clinical applicability of genotyping to tailor antidepressant treatments. A combinatorial categorization approach based on polymorphisms in cytochrome P450 genes (CYP2D6, CYP2C19, CYP2C9, and CYP1A2), SLC6A4 and HTR2A genes, was demonstrated to predict healthcare utilization and disability claims in patients treated with antidepressant drugs. Confirmations and further improvements of this tool are expected to receive recommendation for application in clinical practice according to specific guidelines.

C. Fabbri, MD • A. Serretti, MD, PhD (✉)
Department of Biomedical and Neuromotor Sciences, University of Bologna,
Viale Carlo Pepoli 5, Bologna 40123, Italy
e-mail: chiara.fabbri@yahoo.it; alessandro.serretti@unibo.it

© Springer International Publishing Switzerland 2016
J.K. Rybakowski, A. Serretti (eds.), *Genetic Influences on Response to Drug Treatment for Major Psychiatric Disorders*, DOI 10.1007/978-3-319-27040-1_3

3.1   Introduction

Depressive disorders are responsible for the most part of disability-adjusted life years (DALYs) caused by mental disorders (40.5 %) [48]. Indeed, major depressive disorder (MDD) is associated with morbidity, mortality, and financial costs comparable to other relative common diseases such as hypertension or diabetes [10]. Genetics represents a pivotal research field to understand the biological mechanisms of depression and antidepressant action.

Since the 1990s, the genetic component of antidepressant response has been recognized, thanks to the observation of clustering of this phenotype in families [14]. The following birth of pharmacogenetics provided the possibility of developing an objective tool for guiding antidepressant treatment. Pharmacogenetics (and more recently, pharmacogenomics) is the research field that aims to identify genetic predictors of treatment response and drug-related adverse events, with the aim of improving disease outcome. Indeed, symptom remission during antidepressant treatment is currently reached in only 1/3 of patients, partly due to the lack of effective and reliable predictors of drug response and side effects [14].

The first pharmacogenetic studies were based on the candidate gene approach, i.e., candidate genes were selected a priori on the basis of the known mechanisms of antidepressant action (e.g., monoaminergic genes) and the known molecules involved in antidepressant metabolism.

Given the complex nature of antidepressant action, antidepressant response and side effects are phenotypes affected by a high number of loci with small effect size that presumably interact among each other. Thus, in the first decade of the twenty-first century, genome-wide association studies (GWAS) were developed as attempt to understand the complexity behind these phenotypes, resulting in the birth of pharmacogenomics. The most recent genotyping arrays provide few less than 1,000,000 SNPs throughout the whole genome. GWAS overcome the need of any a priori hypothesis, and they allow to not limit the investigation to individual polymorphisms but extend it to genes and molecular pathways. GWAS have already produced promising results in the study of other complex diseases, such as coronary artery disease, type 1 and 2 diabetes, and rheumatoid arthritis [47], showing to be a powerful method for the detection of genes involved in common human diseases. GWAS focused on antidepressant response and side effects did not report consistent top signals, but some suggestive findings were reported. The lack of consistency among GWAS top signals was probably due to some methodological issues. In particular: (1) the multiple loci with small effect size that are supposed to be involved in antidepressant effect could not be detectable in realistic sample sizes setting alpha error at genome-wide level of significance (i.e. 10^{-8}); (2) phenotypic and genetic heterogeneity within and between samples reduces the chance to reach significance threshold and replicate findings; and (3) previous GWAS mainly focused on individual polymorphisms reducing the chance to replicate findings due to heterogeneity factors. Regarding the latter issue, the focus of genome-wide analyses should be moved from polymorphisms to genes and molecular pathways, since the analysis of functional units is expected to reduce the genetic heterogeneity bias and other sources of heterogeneity among individuals and samples.

In the next paragraphs, the main findings of candidate gene studies and GWAS in the field of antidepressant pharmacogenomics are discussed and linked to the main current hypothesis of antidepressant mechanisms of action. Top genes and polymorphisms are summarized in Table 3.1.

3.1.1 Candidate Gene Studies

3.1.1.1 Monoaminergic System

The monoaminergic theory of MDD was developed from the clinical observation that some compounds, such as iproniazid and imipramine, shared the property of influencing the monoamines' balance in the central nervous system (CNS) and showed unexpected antidepressant effect. On the other hand, reserpine, an old antihypertensive agent that depletes monoamine stores, is able to produce depressive symptoms. Hence, according to the monoaminergic theory, MDD develops as a result of insufficiency of noradrenergic, dopaminergic, and/or serotonergic neurotransmission.

Serotonin Transporter

The serotonin transporter (SERT, encoded by the SLC6A4 gene) regulates serotonin (5-HT) neurotransmission by transporting the neurotransmitter 5-HT from synaptic cleft to presynaptic neurons, and it is the main target of SSRI (selective serotonin reuptake inhibitors) antidepressants.

The most investigated polymorphisms within this gene were the 5-HTTLPR (a 44 bp insertion/deletion), the single nucleotide polymorphism (SNP) rs25531, that are both located in the promoter, and a 17 bp VNTR (variable number of tandem repeats) within intron 2 (STin2).

The 5-HTTLPR 16-repeat sequence is called long allele (L) and it shows a twice basal SERT expression compared to the 11-repeat allele (short allele or S) [14]. The S allele was associated with several psychiatric disorders with affective symptomatology and personality traits related to anxiety, impulsivity, and stress, and with poorer antidepressant response, especially in patients of Caucasian ancestry treated with SSRIs [32]. The S allele was also hypothesized to be a risk factor for SSRI-induced side effects mainly in Caucasian populations, with the exception of sexual side effects [14].

The rs25531 SNP was reported to lay within the 5-HTTLPR sequence and influence the functional effect of 5-HTTLPR itself. Indeed, the rs25531 G variant in conjunction with the L allele (L_G) may result in a reduced expression of SLC6A4, equivalent to that conferred by the S allele [14]. Consistently, single-photon emission computed tomography imaging suggested that L_A/L_A carriers may have a more dynamic serotonergic system that seems to confer higher probability of response to SSRIs. Anyway, pharmacogenetic studies showed substantially negative results [14]. The L_A allele was preliminarily associated with lower SSRI-induced side effects but higher sexual dysfunction in subjects of Caucasian ancestry [17, 22].

Table 3.1 Top findings (replicated by more than two independent studies and/or confirmed by meta-analyses) in antidepressant pharmacogenetics

Gene	Function	Polymorphism(s)	Main finding(s)	Clinical applications	References
SLC6A4	Serotonin transporter	5-HTTLPR	S allele worse response in Caucasians treated with SSRIs and higher risk of SSRI-induced side effects	Included in the GeneSight test	[32, 49]
HTR2A	Serotonin receptor 2A	rs6311; several SNPs in the downstream/first intron region	rs6311 AA worse response in Asians; probable contribution of multiple loci in the downstream/first intron	Included in the GeneSight test	[15, 28, 49]
MAOA	Monoamine catabolism	Promoter VNTR	Worse response in long alleles, possible selective effect in females	/	[14]
COMT	Monoamine catabolism	rs4680 (Val108/158Met)	Met allele better response	/	[14]
GRIK4	Glutamate ionotropic receptor	rs1954787	C allele or CC genotype better response	/	[26]
BDNF	Neurotrophic factor	rs6265 (196G/A or Val66Met)	Heterozygous genotype better response	/	[14, 28]
GNB3	Signal transduction	rs5443 (C825T)	T allele better response	/	[14]
IL-1β	Pro-inflammatory cytokine	rs16944 and rs1143643	G allele of both SNPs worse response	/	[14]
FKBP5	Modulation of glucocorticoid receptor sensitivity	rs3800373	C allele worse response	/	[28]
CYP2D6	Antidepressant metabolism	*1 (wild type), *4, *5, and *10 (alleles with none or decreased activity), gene duplications	Higher treatment efficacy in the intermediate metabolizer group; higher risk of treatment failure in ultrarapid metabolizers; higher side effects in non-extensive metabolizers	Included in the GeneSight test	[16, 49]
CYP2C19	Antidepressant metabolism	*1 (wild type), *2, and *3 (no activity), *17 (increased activity)	Higher side effects in poor metabolizers	Included in the GeneSight test	[16, 49]
ABCB1	Drug efflux pump for xenobiotic compounds in the blood-brain barrier	rs2032582, rs2032583	rs2032582 TT genotype and rs2032583 C allele better response	Preliminary evidence of better outcome in case of genotype-guided treatment compared to treatment as usual	[9, 28]

The STin2 VNTR comprises 9, 10, or 12 copies of a 16–17 bp repeat and may influence gene transcription with a synergistic effect with 5-HTTLPR. Indeed, the 12-repeat variant was shown to cause higher gene expression in vitro and in vivo [14]. Pharmacogenetic findings were mainly negative, while positive results suggested better response in long allele carriers in Asian populations and better response in short allele carriers in Caucasians [14, 25].

Serotonin Receptors

In the field of antidepressant pharmacogenetics, the 5-HT1A (encoded by the HTR1A gene) and 5-HT2A (encoded by the HTR2A gene) serotonin receptor subtypes have been the most investigated.

5-HT1A receptor is abundant in corticolimbic regions, and it could be expressed both pre- and postsynaptically. At the level of serotonin cell bodies in the midbrain, dorsal raphe nucleus acts as an autoreceptor, inhibiting the firing of serotonin neurons and reducing the release of 5-HT in the prefrontal cortex. Antidepressants desensitize these inhibitory autoreceptors and this may be responsible for the delay in antidepressant action onset [46]. On the other hand, reductions in postsynaptic 5-HT1A receptors in prefrontal and temporal cortical regions were demonstrated both in depressive and anxiety disorders [35].

In the HTR1A gene, the most investigated SNP is the rs6295 (or 1019C/G, in the upstream regulatory region of HTR1A), which G allele results in an upregulation of the gene. Thus, rs6295 G allele is expected to contrast the enhancement of serotoninergic transmission through a higher number of presynaptic inhibitory 5-HT1A receptors, resulting in poorer antidepressant response. Nevertheless, pharmacogenetic findings were often inconsistent, and the available meta-analyses suggested no effect of the polymorphism [28]. Different stratification factors were hypothesized to explain these inconsistent findings, in detail: particular subtypes of MDD, gender, or gene x gene interactions [14].

The 5-HT2A receptor is a G-coupled postsynaptic receptor with widespread distribution throughout the cortex, with high densities in the frontal cortex. rs6311 (or -1438A/G) and rs6313 (or 102C/T) are functional HTR2A SNPs in linkage disequilibrium (LD) that have been particularly studied. The rs6313 SNP (within HTR2A exon 1) per se has no likely effect on antidepressant response [28], but gene x gene interactions were suggested to modulate this phenotype or a selective effect on SSRI response was reported [14]. rs6311 is located in the promoter of the gene and the A allele has been associated with increased promoter function [14]. A weak association between the AA genotype and nonresponse in subjects of Asian ancestry was demonstrated [28], but the estimated OR was of only 1.66, with 95 % confidence interval lower limit very close to 1; thus, the detrimental effect of the AA genotype is not more than negligible alone. Anyway, gene x gene interactions involving this locus should not be excluded [14], and additive or multiplicative effects with SNPs within HTR2A or other genes may play relevant effects. Interestingly, the region from the downstream to the first intron of the gene was found to harbor other possibly relevant polymorphisms in the context of antidepressant efficacy. Indeed, rs7333412, rs7324017, rs1923882 [15], and rs7997012 [29] are located in this region and were associated with antidepressant response in a large sample (the Sequenced Treatment Alternatives to Relieve Depression or STAR*D).

Enzymes Responsible for Monoamine Metabolism

The key enzymes involved in the metabolism of monoamines play a role in the regulation of their balance in the CNS.

In regard to serotonin biosynthesis, the limiting step is catalyzed by tryptophan hydroxylase (TPH), which is codified by two distinct genes, TPH1 and TPH2. TPH1 is ubiquitarious but predominantly expressed in peripheral organs, while TPH2 is more selectively expressed in the brain. Anyway, TPH1 and TPH2 are actually expressed at similar levels in some brain areas (e.g., frontal cortex, thalamus, hippocampus, and amygdala), and TPH1 may be selectively expressed in particular circumstances (e.g., stress) [14]. The available pharmacogenetic data are mainly referred to TPH1 rs1800532 (or A218C), because this SNP is located in a potential GATA transcription factor-binding site. The rarer A allele is associated with decreased 5-HT synthesis, and according to the monoaminergic theory of MDD, it may determine worse antidepressant efficacy. The hypothesis was confirmed by some pharmacogenetic studies investigating SSRI response, but the greatest part of them failed to replicate the result [14, 28]. A selective effect of rs1800532 on antidepressant response in specific MDD subtypes (with psychotic and melancholic features) has been recently hypothesized [2], suggesting the usefulness of investigating the SNP in these subgroups of patients. No support to the association between SSRI- and SNRI-induced side effects and rs1800532 was provided [14], a possible effect on antidepressant-induced body weight gain apart [37].

MAO (monoamine oxidase) and COMT (catechol-O-methyltransferase) code for the main enzymes involved in the catabolism of monoamines.

In humans, two distinct MAO isoforms are expressed: MAOA, which is the most investigated one in psychiatry and mainly breaks serotonin, norepinephrine, and epinephrine, and MAOB, which is mainly investigated concerning Parkinson's disease and mainly breaks phenethylamine and benzylamine. A 30-bp VNTR, located 1.2 kb upstream the MAOA coding sequence, was reported to influence the transcription rate of the gene, since alleles with 3.5 or 4 copies of the repeat sequence are transcribed 2–10 times more efficiently than those with 3 or 5 copies of the repeat. Carriers of long alleles were reported to show higher amygdala reactivity in response to aversive stimuli and increase functional coupling of a neural pathway between the ventromedial prefrontal cortex and the amygdala, which was associated to higher levels of harm avoidance, a temperamental dimension related to MDD. Long alleles have been associated with both higher risk of MDD and poorer antidepressant efficacy [30], with a possible selective effect in females [14], consistently with the MAOA position on the X chromosome. Anyway, no all the available studies found an effect of the polymorphism on antidepressant efficacy [14].

The COMT gene is also hypothesized to play a role in MDD pathophysiology and antidepressant response. The COMT Val108/158Met (rs4680) polymorphism shows a relevant functional effect, since the Val/Val genotype catabolizes dopamine at up to four times the rate of Met/Met homozygote, resulting in a significant reduction of synaptic dopamine following neurotransmitter release. Available pharmacogenetic studies mainly reported the Met variant as the favorable allele for antidepressant response, with an allele dose effect (better outcome in Met/Met carriers and intermediate outcome in Met/Val carriers), supporting the monoaminergic theory of MDD. Recently, a better covering of COMT variability was provided, confirming the hypothesis of an effect of this gene on antidepressant efficacy [14].

3.1.1.2   Glutamatergic System

Glutamate is the main excitatory neurotransmitter in the CNS and its effects are mediated both through ionotropic receptors (NMDA, AMPA, and kainate receptors) and receptors that are linked to intracellular second messenger systems (metabotropic or mGlu). Glutamate is hypothesized to affect the risk of MDD and recovery from the disease through neurotoxic and neuroplasticity mechanisms.

The most investigated glutamatergic gene as predictor of antidepressant response is GRIK4 (glutamate receptor, ionotropic, kainate 4), which codes for a member of glutamate kainate receptors responsible for postsynaptic inhibitory neurotransmission. GRIK4 was reported to play a role in the susceptibility to bipolar disorder, schizophrenia and depression, as it has been suggested by the reduced anxiety and antidepressant-like phenotype of the GRIK4(−/−) mice. Pharmacogenetic findings suggested that GRIK4 rs1954787 may affect antidepressant response since patients carrying the C allele or CC genotype were more likely to respond [26].

3.1.1.3   Neuroplasticity

Neurotrophic factors were first characterized for regulating neural growth and differentiation during nervous system development, but are now known to be fundamental regulators of neural plasticity, synaptic plasticity, and neuron survival during adulthood. According to the neurotrophin hypothesis of MDD, a deficiency in neurotrophic support may contribute to the pathogenesis of the disease, and antidepressant drugs may reverse this process [31]. The main genes involved in neurotrophic processes that have been studied in relation to antidepressant pharmacogenetics are BDNF (brain-derived neurotrophic factor) and CREB1 (cyclic AMP response element-binding protein 1). Guanine nucleotide-binding protein (G protein), beta polypeptide 3 (coded by the GNB3 gene), can also be classified as involved in neuroplasticity processes, since the great complexity generated by G proteins in the signal transduction cascade and their large diffusion support the hypothesis that they may contribute to the mechanisms by which neurons acquire the flexibility for generating the wide range of responses observed.

Within the BDNF gene, the rs6265 (196G/A or Val66Met) has been particularly investigated since the Met allele decreases the processing and release of BDNF and is associated with decreased hippocampal volume in humans. Mice with half the normal BDNF (heterozygous deletion mutants) display dendrite deficits and reduced hippocampal volume. Further, they show a phenotype characterized by increased anxiety and reduced response to antidepressants. At functional level, the Met allele was associated with poorer episodic memory and abnormal hippocampal activation [16]. Antidepressant pharmacogenetic studies mainly found a positive molecular heterosis effect of the rs6265, i.e., the heterozygous genotype was associated with better treatment outcome [28]. The result can be explained by animal models showing that although BDNF exerts an antidepressant effect, too high levels may have a detrimental effect on mood [14]. The rs6265 heterozygous genotype advantage observed in antidepressant response may be higher in subjects of Asian ancestry [28], possibly due to the considerable BDNF allele and haplotype diversity among global populations; anyway, some inconsistent or negative findings exist [14].

CREB1 encodes for a transcription factor that is a member of the leucine zipper family of DNA-binding proteins and regulates gene expression, including the induction of BDNF expression. Consistently, increased CREB levels in rodent models result in antidepressant-like behaviors, and studies on both humans and rodents showed that CREB is upregulated by chronic antidepressant treatment [8]. Findings are not unequivocal in regard to the role of CREB1 polymorphisms in antidepressant response. The only replicated finding was the association between rs889895 GG and rs7569963 GG genotypes and remission to antidepressants [12, 38], while different associations were reported by other studies as well as CREB1 x BDNF interactions [27].

The role of the GNB3 rs5443 (C825T) T allele in antidepressant response appears particularly interesting, since this SNP was associated with the occurrence of a splice variant that appears to have altered activity. Four independent studies found that the T allele predicted better antidepressant response, despite opposite or negative findings were reported. Negative findings were all reported in Asian populations, suggesting a possible ethnic stratification effect [14].

3.1.1.4 Inflammation

Inflammation plays a key role in the pathophysiology of MDD and in the mechanisms of antidepressant action. Indeed, (1) one-third of MDD subjects show elevated peripheral inflammatory biomarkers, even in the absence of a medical illness; (2) inflammatory illnesses are associated with greater rates of MDD; (3) patients treated with cytokines (e.g., interferon) are at greater risk of developing MDD; (4) abnormal hypothalamic-pituitary-adrenal (HPA) axis functioning was reported up to the 70 % of patients with MDD; and (5) treatment outcome of MDD is influenced by the antidepressant-induced modulation of cytokines [14].

Cytokines

The most promising pharmacogenetic findings were obtained for interleukin 1β (IL-1β) and interleukin 6 (IL-6). They both code for pro-inflammatory cytokines whose peripheral blood levels were found increased in MDD [16] and inversely correlated with antidepressant response [21]. These cytokines are able to act also within the CNS and affect neuronal death and hippocampal volume [16].

The most interesting polymorphisms within the IL-1β gene are rs16944 and rs1143643. Indeed, functional magnetic resonance imaging showed that the number of G alleles in both rs16944 and rs1143643 was associated with reduced responsiveness of the amygdala and anterior cingulate cortex (ACC) to emotional stimulation [3]. The G allele of both polymorphisms was associated with antidepressant nonresponse [14].

The −174 SNP (rs1800795) within the IL-6 gene is particularly interesting since individuals who carry the G allele have higher plasma concentrations of IL-6 [50], and the polymorphism has been studied as a modulator of interferon (INF)-induced depression [11, 42]. Nevertheless, no data are available about the role of this SNP in antidepressant pharmacological treatment, while the rs7801617 provided a suggestive signal for association with antidepressant response in a GWAS [43].

HPA Axis

Corticotropin-releasing hormone (CRH) receptors 1 and 2 (coded by CRHR1 and CRHR2 genes) are the mediators of the effect of glucocorticoids in the CNS. CRHR1 polymorphisms were hypothesized to modulate antidepressant response particularly in anxious depression as well as in generalized anxiety disorder, while negative results were provided by some studies that did not consider anxiety levels [14]. High anxiety-related behavior mice show altered expression of the CRHR1 gene in the pituitary and prefrontal cortex [39]. Furthermore, CRHR1 system is implicated in the programming effects of early life stress on eventual anxious-depressive psychopathology [45]. Few and non-replicated findings are available for the CRHR2 gene as well as for the NR3C1 gene (coding for the glucocorticoid receptor or GR) [14].

The FKBP5 (FK506-binding protein 52) acts as a cochaperon for GR maturation, modulating its sensitivity and thus playing a role in regulation of stress response. Indeed, increased expression of the FKBP5 gene confers elevated GR resistance [6], and glucocorticoids induce FKBP5 expression. Chronic antidepressant treatment is able to normalize such alterations [20]. Despite negative pharmacogenetic findings that were reported for this gene [14], meta-analytic results supported the effect of rs3800373 on antidepressant response in subjects of Caucasian ethnicity [28] as well as the studies on the largest sample sizes reported that rs1360780, rs3800373, rs4713916, and rs352428 may modulate antidepressant response. Interestingly, rs1360780 TT genotype was associated with faster response, modulation of FKBP5 expression, and a faster restoration of normal HPA-axis function [7].

3.1.1.5 Antidepressant Pharmacokinetics

The enzymes involved in antidepressant metabolism, clearance, and transport are hypothesized to play a relevant role in interindividual differences observed in antidepressant efficacy and side effects. Particularly, the enzymes coded by cytochrome P450 (CYP) and ABCB1 genes (P-glycoprotein) are mainly responsible for antidepressant transport and metabolism [33].

Cytochrome P450 Genes

The cytochrome P450 (CYP) superfamily is the major enzyme class responsible for the oxidation and reduction of numerous organic substrates, including drugs. The isoenzymes mainly involved in antidepressant metabolism are CYP2D6, CYP2C19, CYP2C9, and CYP2B6, which coding genes are highly polymorphic. Alleles at polymorphic loci within these genes can show normal, partially or totally defective activity, defining some theoretical metabolizing groups according to the allele combination [33].

The metabolizing group shows a well-documented association with antidepressant pharmacokinetic measures, and theoretical dose adjustments were determined accordingly. Pharmacogenetic studies focused on the association between metabolizing status and antidepressant response often provided inconsistent findings [33]. The most robust finding was the association between CYP2D6 metabolizing activity and response to several antidepressants. In detail, higher response rate was reported in CYP2D6 intermediate metabolizers (IMs), and higher risk of treatment failure and suicide was associated with CYP2D6 ultrarapid metabolizer (UM) status. Regarding tolerability, higher occurrence/severity of side effects was reported in non-extensive CYP2D6 or CYP2C19 metabolizers [16].

ABCB1 Gene

P-glycoprotein (P-gp, coded by the ABCB1 gene) is an ATP-dependent drug efflux pump for xenobiotic compounds that decreases drug accumulation in multidrug resistant cells and limits the uptake of drugs into key organs such as the brain. Animal studies showed that a wide variety of structurally unrelated drugs are efficaciously carried out from the brain, thanks to P-gp activity, among which a number of antidepressants, with some exceptions (fluoxetine, bupropion, mirtazapine) [14].

The ABCB1 SNPs rs2032582 (G2677) and rs1045642 (3435C) were associated with altered P-gp expression and function. Some previous studies demonstrated an effect of rs2032582 and rs1045642 on antidepressant response, and the effect of rs2032582 was confirmed by a meta-analysis [28]. Further studies suggested that also rs2032583 and rs2235040 may be genetic modulators of response, but the association is depending from being or not the prescribed antidepressant a P-gp substrate [16]. Interestingly, the rs2232583 SNP may be involved in resistance to antidepressant treatment: the TT genotype was hypothesized to increase drug export out of the brain, requiring dose adjustment or switch to a drug which is not a substrate of P-gp [34, 44]. Regarding antidepressant-induced side effects, the A allele of the rs2032588 SNP was associated with a lower number of side effects only in P-gp-dependent antidepressant users [4]; as well as the functional rs10245483 may impact on side-effect ratings but depending from the used antidepressant [36].

3.1.2   Genome-Wide Association Studies (GWAS)

GWAS provided interesting findings concerning both individual genes and molecular pathways that may be implicated in antidepressant response. Despite they did not reach the stringent p threshold for genome-wide significance (10^{-8}), signals within the RORA (RAR-related orphan receptor A) [18], IL-11, IL-6 [43], and NRG1 (neuregulin-1) [5] genes were the top findings considering both the strength of association with antidepressant response and the biological function of their products. RORA is involved in the regulation of the circadian rhythm (which is highly disrupted in MDD) and it was correlated with trait depression at genome-wide level [14]. IL-11 and IL-6 genes code for interleukins, and their involvement in MDD and mechanisms of antidepressant action is highly supported by the inflammation theory of depression (see Sect. 3.1.1.4). NRG1 is involved in many aspects of brain development, including neuronal maturation, and variations in this gene have been shown to be associated with increased risk for mental disorders [5].

The available genome-wide response data from several samples were further analyzed together by means of meta-analyses, but neither individual marker reached the significance threshold nor promising trends were reported [19, 41]. Among the possible reasons for these negative findings, clinical and genetic heterogeneity among the included samples may have played a role. On the other hand, multilocus analysis and pathway analysis (i.e., the analysis of the combined effect of a number of top SNPs in different genes, possibly in the same molecular pathway) provided more encouraging results, probably because the investigation of cluster of interrelated polymorphisms instead of individual polymorphisms reduces the heterogeneity bias. Indeed, a multilocus analysis across two GWAS found that response was positively affected by a number of common alleles and top genes could be grouped in three main molecular clusters (metabolic pathways and brain development, metabolic and cardiovascular diseases, GABAergic and glutamatergic neurotransmission) [24]. Pathway analyses of genome-wide data found that pathways involved in inflammation (B-cell receptor signaling pathway [15], antigen-processing and presentation pathway, tumor necrosis factor pathway [23]), and neural plasticity (long-term potentiation pathway [23] and GAP43 pathway [13]) are significantly involved in the modulation of antidepressant efficacy.

3.2 Clinical Applicability

The study of clinical outcomes and cost/benefit ratio of genotyping to guide antidepressant treatments is fundamental to evaluate clinical applicability. A pharmacogenetic test (GeneSight) based on polymorphisms in cytochrome P450 genes (CYP2D6, CYP2C19, CYP2C9, and CYP1A2), SLC6A4, and HTR2A genes has showed a positive impact on healthcare utilization measures. Indeed, an evident increase of healthcare utilization measures was demonstrated in patients who were identified by the gene-based interpretive report as most at risk for the prescribed medication regimen. These patients had 69 % more total healthcare visits and greater than threefold more medical absence days than subjects taking drugs categorized by the gene-based report as with no risk or intermediate risk [49]. These findings have been confirmed by following analyses, supporting that the combinatorial categorization approach of the GeneSight test discriminates and predicts healthcare utilization and disability claims, while individual genes were not able to predict these outcomes [1]. In addition to the GeneSight test, clinical outcomes of a genotype-guided treatment based on ABCB1 rs2032583 and rs2235015 SNPs were investigated in comparison with treatment as usual. Differences in choice of treatment strategies were applied after the receipt of the ABCB1 test result in the genotype-guided arm. Patients who received ABCB1 genotyping had higher remission rates and lower symptom severity at the time of discharge from hospital as compared to patients without ABCB1 testing [9].

3.3 Conclusion

A number of genes involved in the pharmacokinetics and pharmacodynamics of antidepressants is expected to contribute to treatment outcomes. Indeed, the variance in antidepressant response due to a single variant is estimated to be low (e.g., not more than 3.2 % for 5-HTTLPR [14]), and pharmacogenetic tests aimed to predict antidepressant response are expected to combine different loci, probably in different genes, such as the GeneSight test (see Sect. 3.2). Anyway, a better definition of the genes and molecular pathways involved in antidepressant action is needed for the development and optimization of tests suitable for clinical practice. Pharmacogenetic studies have demonstrated a number of limitations, both specific of this kind of study (see Sect. 3.1) and common to other types of trial (e.g., insufficient statistical power, inadequate inclusion criteria often resulting in clinical heterogeneity, use of mixed medication regimens). The quality of research in this field has shown a great improvement in the last years, due to the efforts that have been made to improve the personal and social burden of MDD. Indeed, the establishment of consortiums (e.g., major depressive disorder working group of the psychiatric GWAS Consortium) aimed to enlarge available samples and improve the applied analysis tools has recently became a new horizon in the field. Thus, large GWAS meta-analysis, GWAS pathway analysis, and the attempt to define more homogeneous phenotypes have been performed. Genome-wide data analysis confirmed the relevance of common SNP contribution to antidepressant response, estimating that they explain 42 % of individual differences in antidepressant response [40]. These recent improvements get an encouraging perspective on the future development of antidepressant pharmacogenetics.

References

1. Altar CA, Carhart JM, Allen JD, Hall-Flavin DK, Dechairo BM, Winner JG (2015) Clinical validity: combinatorial pharmacogenomics predicts antidepressant responses and healthcare utilizations better than single gene phenotypes. Pharmacogenomics J. doi:10.1038/tpj.2014.85
2. Arias B, Fabbri C, Gressier F, Serretti A, Mitjans M, Gasto C, Catalan R, De Ronchi D, Fananas L (2013) TPH1, MAOA, serotonin receptor 2A and 2C genes in citalopram response: possible effect in melancholic and psychotic depression. Neuropsychobiology 67(1):41–47. doi:10.1159/000343388
3. Baune BT, Dannlowski U, Domschke K, Janssen DG, Jordan MA, Ohrmann P, Bauer J, Biros E, Arolt V, Kugel H, Baxter AG, Suslow T (2010) The interleukin 1 beta (IL1B) gene is associated with failure to achieve remission and impaired emotion processing in major depression. Biol Psychiatry 67(6):543–549. doi:10.1016/j.biopsych.2009.11.004
4. Bet PM, Verbeek EC, Milaneschi Y, Straver DB, Uithuisje T, Bevova MR, Hugtenburg JG, Heutink P, Penninx BW, Hoogendijk WJ (2015) A common polymorphism in the ABCB1 gene is associated with side effects of PGP-dependent antidepressants in a large naturalistic Dutch cohort. Pharmacogenomics J. doi:10.1038/tpj.2015.38
5. Biernacka JM, Sangkuhl K, Jenkins G, Whaley RM, Barman P, Batzler A, Altman RB, Arolt V, Brockmoller J, Chen CH, Domschke K, Hall-Flavin DK, Hong CJ, Illi A, Ji Y, Kampman O, Kinoshita T, Leinonen E, Liou YJ, Mushiroda T, Nonen S, Skime MK, Wang L, Baune BT, Kato M, Liu YL, Praphanphoj V, Stingl JC, Tsai SJ, Kubo M, Klein TE, Weinshilboum R (2015) The International SSRI Pharmacogenomics Consortium (ISPC): a genome-wide association study of antidepressant treatment response. Transl Psychiatry 5:e553. doi:10.1038/tp.2015.47
6. Binder EB (2009) The role of FKBP5, a co-chaperone of the glucocorticoid receptor in the pathogenesis and therapy of affective and anxiety disorders. Psychoneuroendocrinology 34(Suppl 1):S186–S195. doi:10.1016/j.psyneuen.2009.05.021
7. Binder EB, Salyakina D, Lichtner P, Wochnik GM, Ising M, Putz B, Papiol S, Seaman S, Lucae S, Kohli MA, Nickel T, Kunzel HE, Fuchs B, Majer M, Pfennig A, Kern N, Brunner J, Modell S, Baghai T, Deiml T, Zill P, Bondy B, Rupprecht R, Messer T, Kohnlein O, Dabitz H, Bruckl T, Muller N, Pfister H, Lieb R, Mueller JC, Lohmussaar E, Strom TM, Bettecken T, Meitinger T, Uhr M, Rein T, Holsboer F, Muller-Myhsok B (2004) Polymorphisms in FKBP5 are associated with increased recurrence of depressive episodes and rapid response to antidepressant treatment. Nat Genet 36(12):1319–1325. doi:10.1038/ng1479
8. Blendy JA (2006) The role of CREB in depression and antidepressant treatment. Biol Psychiatry 59(12):1144–1150

9. Breitenstein B, Scheuer S, Pfister H, Uhr M, Lucae S, Holsboer F, Ising M, Bruckl TM (2014) The clinical application of ABCB1 genotyping in antidepressant treatment: a pilot study. CNS Spectr 19(2):165–175. doi:10.1017/S1092852913000436

10. Buist-Bouwman MA, De Graaf R, Vollebergh WA, Alonso J, Bruffaerts R, Ormel J (2006) Functional disability of mental disorders and comparison with physical disorders: a study among the general population of six European countries. Acta Psychiatr Scand 113(6):492–500

11. Bull SJ, Huezo-Diaz P, Binder EB, Cubells JF, Ranjith G, Maddock C, Miyazaki C, Alexander N, Hotopf M, Cleare AJ, Norris S, Cassidy E, Aitchison KJ, Miller AH, Pariante CM (2009) Functional polymorphisms in the interleukin-6 and serotonin transporter genes, and depression and fatigue induced by interferon-alpha and ribavirin treatment. Mol Psychiatry 14(12):1095–1104. doi:10.1038/mp.2008.48

12. Calati R, Crisafulli C, Balestri M, Serretti A, Spina E, Calabro M, Sidoti A, Albani D, Massat I, Hofer P, Amital D, Juven-Wetzler A, Kasper S, Zohar J, Souery D, Montgomery S, Mendlewicz J (2013) Evaluation of the role of MAPK1 and CREB1 polymorphisms on treatment resistance, response and remission in mood disorder patients. Prog Neuropsychopharmacol Biol Psychiatry 44:271–278. doi:10.1016/j.pnpbp.2013.03.005

13. Fabbri C, Crisafulli C, Gurwitz D, Stingl J, Calati R, Albani D, Forloni G, Calabrò M, Martines R, Kasper S, Zohar J, Juven-Wetzler A, Souery D, Montgomery S, Mendlewicz J, De Girolamo G, Serretti A (2015) Neuronal cell adhesion genes and antidepressant response in three independent samples. Pharmacogenomics J 15(6):538–548

14. Fabbri C, Di Girolamo G, Serretti A (2013) Pharmacogenetics of antidepressant drugs: an update after almost 20 years of research. Am J Med Genet B Neuropsychiatr Genet 162B(6):487–520. doi:10.1002/ajmg.b.32184

15. Fabbri C, Marsano A, Albani D, Chierchia A, Calati R, Drago A, Crisafulli C, Calabro M, Kasper S, Lanzenberger R, Zohar J, Juven-Wetzler A, Souery D, Montgomery S, Mendlewicz J, Serretti A (2014) PPP3CC gene: a putative modulator of antidepressant response through the B-cell receptor signaling pathway. Pharmacogenomics J 14(5):463–472. doi:10.1038/tpj.2014.15

16. Fabbri C, Serretti A (2015) Pharmacogenetics of major depressive disorder: top genes and pathways toward clinical applications. Curr Psychiatry Rep 17(7):594. doi:10.1007/s11920-015-0594-9

17. Garfield LD, Dixon D, Nowotny P, Lotrich FE, Pollock BG, Kristjansson SD, Dore PM, Lenze EJ (2014) Common selective serotonin reuptake inhibitor side effects in older adults associated with genetic polymorphisms in the serotonin transporter and receptors: data from a randomized controlled trial. Am J Geriatr Psychiatry 22(10):971–979. doi:10.1016/j.jagp.2013.07.003

18. Garriock HA, Kraft JB, Shyn SI, Peters EJ, Yokoyama JS, Jenkins GD, Reinalda MS, Slager SL, McGrath PJ, Hamilton SP (2010) A genomewide association study of citalopram response in major depressive disorder. Biol Psychiatry 67(2):133–138. doi:10.1016/j.biopsych.2009.08.029

19. GENDEP Investigators; MARS Investigators; STAR*D Investigators (2013) Common genetic variation and antidepressant efficacy in major depressive disorder: a meta-analysis of three genome-wide pharmacogenetic studies. Am J Psychiatry 170(2):207–217. doi:10.1176/appi.ajp.2012.12020237

20. Guidotti G, Calabrese F, Anacker C, Racagni G, Pariante CM, Riva MA (2013) Glucocorticoid receptor and FKBP5 expression is altered following exposure to chronic stress: modulation by antidepressant treatment. Neuropsychopharmacology 38(4):616–627. doi:10.1038/npp.2012.225

21. Hannestad J, DellaGioia N, Bloch M (2011) The effect of antidepressant medication treatment on serum levels of inflammatory cytokines: a meta-analysis. Neuropsychopharmacology 36(12):2452–2459. doi:10.1038/npp.2011.132

22. Hu XZ, Rush AJ, Charney D, Wilson AF, Sorant AJ, Papanicolaou GJ, Fava M, Trivedi MH, Wisniewski SR, Laje G, Paddock S, McMahon FJ, Manji H, Lipsky RH (2007) Association

between a functional serotonin transporter promoter polymorphism and citalopram treatment in adult outpatients with major depression. Arch Gen Psychiatry 64(7):783–792

23. Hunter AM, Leuchter AF, Power RA, Muthen B, McGrath PJ, Lewis CM, Cook IA, Garriock HA, McGuffin P, Uher R, Hamilton SP (2013) A genome-wide association study of a sustained pattern of antidepressant response. J Psychiatr Res 47(9):1157–1165. doi:10.1016/j.jpsychires.2013.05.002

24. Ising M, Lucae S, Binder EB, Bettecken T, Uhr M, Ripke S, Kohli MA, Hennings JM, Horstmann S, Kloiber S, Menke A, Bondy B, Rupprecht R, Domschke K, Baune BT, Arolt V, Rush AJ, Holsboer F, Muller-Myhsok B (2009) A genomewide association study points to multiple loci that predict antidepressant drug treatment outcome in depression. Arch Gen Psychiatry 66(9):966–975

25. Kato M, Serretti A (2010) Review and meta-analysis of antidepressant pharmacogenetic findings in major depressive disorder. Mol Psychiatry 15(5):473–500

26. Kawaguchi DM, Glatt SJ (2014) GRIK4 polymorphism and its association with antidepressant response in depressed patients: a meta-analysis. Pharmacogenomics 15(11):1451–1459. doi:10.2217/pgs.14.96

27. Murphy GM Jr, Hollander SB, Rodrigues HE, Kremer C, Schatzberg AF (2004) Effects of the serotonin transporter gene promoter polymorphism on mirtazapine and paroxetine efficacy and adverse events in geriatric major depression. Arch Gen Psychiatry 61(11):1163–1169

28. Niitsu T, Fabbri C, Bentini F, Serretti A (2013) Pharmacogenetics in major depression: a comprehensive meta-analysis. Prog Neuropsychopharmacol Biol Psychiatry 45:183–194. doi:10.1016/j.pnpbp.2013.05.011

29. Peters EJ, Slager SL, Jenkins GD, Reinalda MS, Garriock HA, Shyn SI, Kraft JB, McGrath PJ, Hamilton SP (2009) Resequencing of serotonin-related genes and association of tagging SNPs to citalopram response. Pharmacogenet Genomics 19(1):1–10

30. Porcelli S, Drago A, Fabbri C, Gibiino S, Calati R, Serretti A (2011) Pharmacogenetics of antidepressant response. J Psychiatry Neurosci 36(2):87–113

31. Porcelli S, Drago A, Fabbri C, Serretti A (2011) Mechanisms of antidepressant action: an integrated dopaminergic perspective. Prog Neuropsychopharmacol Biol Psychiatry 35(7):1532–1543

32. Porcelli S, Fabbri C, Serretti A (2012) Meta-analysis of serotonin transporter gene promoter polymorphism (5-HTTLPR) association with antidepressant efficacy. Eur Neuropsychopharmacol 22(4):239–258

33. Porcelli S, Fabbri C, Spina E, Serretti A, De Ronchi D (2011) Genetic polymorphisms of cytochrome P450 enzymes and antidepressant metabolism. Expert Opin Drug Metab Toxicol 7(9):1101–1115

34. Rosenhagen MC, Uhr M (2010) Single nucleotide polymorphism in the drug transporter gene ABCB1 in treatment-resistant depression: clinical practice. J Clin Psychopharmacol 30(2):209–211

35. Savitz J, Lucki I, Drevets WC (2009) 5-HT(1A) receptor function in major depressive disorder. Prog Neurobiol 88(1):17–31. doi:10.1016/j.pneurobio.2009.01.009

36. Schatzberg AF, DeBattista C, Lazzeroni LC, Etkin A, Murphy GM Jr, Williams LM (2015) ABCB1 genetic effects on antidepressant outcomes: a report from the iSPOT-D trial. Am J Psychiatry. doi:10.1176/appi.ajp.2015.14050680

37. Secher A, Bukh J, Bock C, Koefoed P, Rasmussen HB, Werge T, Kessing LV, Mellerup E (2009) Antidepressive-drug-induced bodyweight gain is associated with polymorphisms in genes coding for COMT and TPH1. Int Clin Psychopharmacol 24(4):199–203. doi:10.1097/YIC.0b013e32832d6be2

38. Serretti A, Chiesa A, Calati R, Massat I, Linotte S, Kasper S, Lecrubier Y, Antonijevic I, Forray C, Snyder L, Bollen J, Zohar J, De Ronchi D, Souery D, Mendlewicz J (2011) A preliminary investigation of the influence of CREB1 gene on treatment resistance in major depression. J Affect Disord 128(1–2):56–63. doi:10.1016/j.jad.2010.06.025

39. Sotnikov S, Wittmann A, Bunck M, Bauer S, Deussing J, Schmidt M, Touma C, Landgraf R, Czibere L (2014) Blunted HPA axis reactivity reveals glucocorticoid system dysbalance in a

mouse model of high anxiety-related behavior. Psychoneuroendocrinology 48:41–51. doi:10.1016/j.psyneuen.2014.06.006

40. Tansey KE, Guipponi M, Hu X, Domenici E, Lewis G, Malafosse A, Wendland JR, Lewis CM, McGuffin P, Uher R (2013) Contribution of common genetic variants to antidepressant response. Biol Psychiatry 73(7):679–682. doi:10.1016/j.biopsych.2012.10.030

41. Tansey KE, Guipponi M, Perroud N, Bondolfi G, Domenici E, Evans D, Hall SK, Hauser J, Henigsberg N, Hu X, Jerman B, Maier W, Mors O, O'Donovan M, Peters TJ, Placentino A, Rietschel M, Souery D, Aitchison KJ, Craig I, Farmer A, Wendland JR, Malafosse A, Holmans P, Lewis G, Lewis CM, Stensbol TB, Kapur S, McGuffin P, Uher R (2012) Genetic predictors of response to serotonergic and noradrenergic antidepressants in major depressive disorder: a genome-wide analysis of individual-level data and a meta-analysis. PLoS Med 9(10):e1001326. doi:10.1371/journal.pmed.1001326

42. Udina M, Moreno-Espana J, Navines R, Gimenez D, Langohr K, Gratacos M, Capuron L, de la Torre R, Sola R, Martin-Santos R (2013) Serotonin and interleukin-6: the role of genetic polymorphisms in IFN-induced neuropsychiatric symptoms. Psychoneuroendocrinology 38(9):1803–1813. doi:10.1016/j.psyneuen.2013.03.007

43. Uher R, Perroud N, Ng MY, Hauser J, Henigsberg N, Maier W, Mors O, Placentino A, Rietschel M, Souery D, Zagar T, Czerski PM, Jerman B, Larsen ER, Schulze TG, Zobel A, Cohen-Woods S, Pirlo K, Butler AW, Muglia P, Barnes MR, Lathrop M, Farmer A, Breen G, Aitchison KJ, Craig I, Lewis CM, McGuffin P (2010) Genome-wide pharmacogenetics of antidepressant response in the GENDEP project. Am J Psychiatry 167(5):555–564. doi:10.1176/appi.ajp.2009.09070932

44. Uhr M, Tontsch A, Namendorf C, Ripke S, Lucae S, Ising M, Dose T, Ebinger M, Rosenhagen M, Kohli M, Kloiber S, Salyakina D, Bettecken T, Specht M, Putz B, Binder EB, Muller-Myhsok B, Holsboer F (2008) Polymorphisms in the drug transporter gene ABCB1 predict antidepressant treatment response in depression. Neuron 57(2):203–209

45. Veenit V, Riccio O, Sandi C (2014) CRHR1 links peripuberty stress with deficits in social and stress-coping behaviors. J Psychiatr Res 53:1–7. doi:10.1016/j.jpsychires.2014.02.015

46. Watson JM, Dawson LA (2007) Characterization of the potent 5-HT(1A/B) receptor antagonist and serotonin reuptake inhibitor SB-649915: preclinical evidence for hastened onset of antidepressant/anxiolytic efficacy. CNS Drug Rev 13(2):206–223. doi:10.1111/j.1527-3458.2007.00012.x

47. Wellcome Trust Case Control Consortium (2007) Genome-wide association study of 14,000 cases of seven common diseases and 3,000 shared controls. Nature 447(7145):661–678

48. Whiteford HA, Degenhardt L, Rehm J, Baxter AJ, Ferrari AJ, Erskine HE, Charlson FJ, Norman RE, Flaxman AD, Johns N, Burstein R, Murray CJ, Vos T (2013) Global burden of disease attributable to mental and substance use disorders: findings from the Global Burden of Disease Study 2010. Lancet 382(9904):1575–1586. doi:10.1016/S0140-6736(13)61611-6

49. Winner J, Allen JD, Altar CA, Spahic-Mihajlovic A (2013) Psychiatric pharmacogenomics predicts health resource utilization of outpatients with anxiety and depression. Transl Psychiatry 3:e242. doi:10.1038/tp.2013.2

50. Zakharyan R, Petrek M, Arakelyan A, Mrazek F, Atshemyan S, Boyajyan A (2012) Interleukin-6 promoter polymorphism and plasma levels in patients with schizophrenia. Tissue Antigens 80(2):136–142. doi:10.1111/j.1399-0039.2012.01886.x

Chapter 4
Genomic Studies of Treatment Resistance in Major Depressive Disorder

Roy H. Perlis

Abstract Treatment-resistant depression describes the subset of individuals with major depressive disorder who do not reach symptomatic remission despite multiple adequate treatment trials. While treatment resistance has a substantial impact on functioning, quality of life, and healthcare costs, little is known about the underlying neurobiology. While at least some treatment-resistant depression (TRD) risk is likely to be heritable, based primarily on evidence from antidepressant pharmacogenomics, studies to date have failed to reliably identify rare or common genetic variation associated with this phenotype. Challenges in the study of TRD include misclassification arising from medication intolerance or inadequate treatment trials, the heterogeneity of the concept itself, and most notably the absence of well-characterized cohorts with DNA available for study. New strategies to identify large cohorts from biobanks or disease registries and efforts to meta-analyze multiple cohorts may facilitate the identification of risk variants. In addition, further studies to understand the potential utility of pharmacogenomic testing among individuals with TRD or to stratify risk for TRD are needed.

4.1 Background and Motivation

Around 1/3 of individuals who receive initial antidepressant treatment for major depressive disorder will not reach symptomatic remission. A subset of these, perhaps approaching 50 %, will not remit despite additional antidepressant treatment [31]. Such nonremission in the face of adequate antidepressant trials is referred to as treatment-resistant depression [9], a concept first characterized more than 40

R.H. Perlis, MD, MSc
Department of Psychiatry and the Center for Human Genetic Research,
Center for Experimental Drugs and Diagnostics, Massachusetts General Hospital,
Boston, MA 02114, USA
e-mail: rperlis@partners.org

© Springer International Publishing Switzerland 2016
J.K. Rybakowski, A. Serretti (eds.), *Genetic Influences on Response to Drug Treatment for Major Psychiatric Disorders*, DOI 10.1007/978-3-319-27040-1_4

55

years ago [15]. Both the retrospective assessment of antidepressant treatment history [24, 37] and the definition of treatment resistance itself have varied. In general, however, treatment-resistant depression is often taken to refer to the absence of remission following at least two adequate treatment trials in the current episode. (While past definitions often required two trials of medications of different classes, more recently even two SSRI failures may be considered TRD, on the basis of evidence from studies such as STAR*D suggesting similar probability of response to next-step treatment regardless of medication class [31].

The clinical rationale for studying treatment resistance relates to the consequences of more prolonged depression: a longer period of vulnerability to suicide, functional impairment, and poorer quality of life. Treatment-resistant depression makes a major contribution to the cost of depression as a whole: directly, by consuming more treatment resources and, indirectly, by increasing the cost of other comorbidities across medicine. For example, one claims study found medical costs 40 % greater among individuals with TRD [13].

Pharmacogenomics is often tied to personalized medicine, the effort to match individuals to treatment most effective for them. In the case of TRD, however, even stratified medicine – achieving more precise estimates of risk for multiple treatment failures, even where the specific effective treatment cannot yet be predicted – could have profound public health implications.

4.2   Rationale for Genetic Investigation

Standard approaches to establishing the genetic basis for a disease relied on family and twin investigations. For antidepressant response, because of changes in treatment, in frequency of diagnosis, and in definitions of depression itself, such studies have been extremely sparse. For antidepressant response in general, there is modest evidence from family studies [11, 23, 25] and a twin study [1].

A more modern methodology examines genome-wide association data to estimate the extent to which a phenotype is heritable Genome-wide Complex Trait Analysis (GCTA). Applied to antidepressant response, this approach yields estimates up to ~42 %, a figure which substantially exceeds that of MDD itself [35] However, the very large confidence interval around this estimate renders the point estimate difficult to interpret, so establishing the actual heritability of antidepressant response awaits larger patient samples.

In this context, it is not surprising that there is essentially no evidence that TRD – a phenotype even more difficult to characterize in families, twin studies, or large cohorts – is likely to be genetic. Indeed, as discussed later in this chapter, there are numerous contributors to apparent TRD that are not genetic or at least not specific for TRD. However, there are at least three indirect lines of evidence that suggest that it is reasonable to investigate TRD.

First, as we have noted, there is modest evidence for the familiality and heritability of antidepressant response, which might be expected to represent a lower boundary for inherited risk for TRD, a more extreme phenotype. Second, animal models suggest that genetic variation may influence responsiveness to antidepressants. In particular, rodent quantitative trait studies suggest loci such as vesicular monoamine transporter 2 (VMAT2, or slc18a2) associated with differential antidepressant effects [7].

A third argument is largely theoretical. Antidepressants of multiple mechanisms have demonstrated effectiveness in MDD. A broad range of monoaminergic antidepressants exhibit efficacy – while serotonin reuptake has been a focus on the basis of selective serotonin reuptake inhibitors, older antidepressants and some newer ones exhibit noradrenergic and dopaminergic mechanisms. (Indeed, the antidepressant tianeptine is characterized as enhancing rather than inhibiting serotonin reuptake.) Most recently, the efficacy of glutamatergic antidepressants such as ketamine provides clear evidence for the complexity of treatment response [43].

In many biological pathways, stimuli of different types may converge on one or a few key proteins, such as kinases, before effecting a response. While blocking any individual stimulus may still allow response, knocking out a critical element may eliminate responsiveness. Extending this argument to antidepressants suggests that, despite their multiple proximal mechanisms, they may converge on common elements to mediate antidepressant response. (An alternate model posits multiple mechanisms for MDD itself, such that certain antidepressants work only for one or a few mechanisms; under this model, predicting treatment response would require identification of the features that identify each mechanism or subtype.) If this is the case, TRD could arise from variations that influence signaling upstream from antidepressant proximal site of action, thereby affecting response to multiple antidepressant types though not necessarily all of them.

Beyond these three arguments for the plausibility of treatment resistance genetics lies a more general rationale for investigating this category of treatment outcomes. In particular, basic statistics suggests that studying more extreme phenotypes may yield greater power to detect associations, per observation, than studying all phenotypes jointly. Such outliers may have a larger "dose" of genetic risk or individual risk variants of larger effect, rendering them easier to detect.

For antidepressant response, the substantial rates of placebo response and inability to reliably distinguish these responses from true drug response may render it difficult to detect extremely positive response. On the other hand, extremely poor antidepressant response is a more extreme phenotype than single treatment failure. Thus, focusing on these individuals may allow greater power to detect risk variants. (Indeed, the possibility that studies of SSRI response may really represent studies of placebo response represents another rationale for focusing on treatment resistance; antidepressant-placebo differences in large meta-analyses are typically modest [10].)

4.3   Association Studies of TRD

Based upon a PubMed search of genetic association, treatment resistance, and major depressive disorder, as well as common synonyms, only one published study has examined treatment resistance in an unbiased or genome-wide fashion. In that investigation, the author and colleagues utilized electronic health records to identify a cohort of 300 individuals who had not responded to at least two adequate antidepressant trials and contrasted them to 478 who responded to an initial SSRI trial. Hypothesizing that rarer deleterious variants – i.e., copy number variation – might exert larger and thus more detectable effects in aggregate than single nucleotide polymorphisms, we sought to identify genes with greater burden of copy number variants among TRD patients compared to controls.

That study further examined 485 individuals from the Sequenced Treatment Alternatives to Relieve Depression (STAR*D) cohort, contrasting 152 who prospectively did not respond to two or more treatments with 333 SSRI-responsive individuals.

Overall, a modest increase in duplicated DNA regions in the 100–200 kilobase range was observed among TRD individuals. No individual loci reached a genome-wide threshold for association with TRD, although one deletion spanning PABPC4L was observed in six cases and no controls. While promising, this result underscores one of the challenges in studying TRD: because the cohorts are difficult to collect and characterize, there is a paucity of such samples available, so replication has not been possible. (A second study, using the NEWMEDS cohort, also examined copy number variation, but focused on overall antidepressant response rather than treatment resistance [36]; evidence of enrichment of duplications was not observed.)

To date, there are no published genome-wide studies examining common variation in TRD, although several candidate gene-based studies have appeared. These are in general very difficult to interpret for multiple reasons. First, and most importantly, these studies include very small treatment cohorts – in most cases, one to two orders of magnitude smaller than modern GWAS investigations. As such, the risk for false negatives is extremely high for all but the largest effects. Further, many studies examined only a single SNP or a small number of SNPs in one or a few genes; this limits the risk of false positives arising from multiple comparisons, but does not exclude the possibility that other variations in the genes studied do have real effects. Third, most studies made no effort to address population stratification, apart from restricting analysis to self-reported ethnicity, so the risk for stratification artifact is high. Finally, for some cohorts, each individual association study was reported separately, without consideration of or correction for the number of genes previously investigated.

Perhaps the greatest challenge in such candidate-based studies is the paucity of plausible candidates given the very poor understanding of the underlying neurobiology of treatment resistance. Certainly the most plausible candidates may be drawn from the genes which code the major metabolic enzymes for which antidepressants are substrates, those of the cytochrome p450 (CYP450) system. The evidence that these variants are important for antidepressants is strongest for tricyclic antidepressants but mixed for SSRIs and other newer agents [26].

On the basis of an admittedly weak relationship between CYP450 phenotypes and blood levels, one could hypothesize that individuals with duplications of CYP450 enzymes leading to increased function – so-called ultrarapid metabolizers – might be overrepresented among TRD individuals, as they might fail to respond because of an inability to achieve therapeutic blood levels. Surprisingly, this has never been tested in a large cohort of TRD subjects. In one study of 55 individuals who had failed to respond to two CYP450 2D6 antidepressants, no enrichment of ultrarapid metabolizers (<2 % of the cohort, as well as the reference population) was observed [14].

Alternatively, one might hypothesize that less efficient metabolizers – poor metabolizers – would be enriched in light of inability to tolerate standard antidepressant doses. This, too, has not been systematically investigated apart from the small study of Haber et al, which observed a prevalence of 14.5 % for poor metabolizers, somewhat higher than the anticipated 8.3 % but not significantly so.

One of the first investigations of TRD [29] examined four genes that had been suggested in rodent models of antidepressant response and characterized the STAR*D cohort [see Chap. [3]] not in terms of citalopram response, but in terms of level 2 and 3 (i.e., next-step) treatment outcomes. Of the four genes studied, one – the potassium channel gene KCNK2, or TREK1 – was significantly associated with failure to respond to two or more treatments and three or more treatments in STAR*D. Notably, this effect was not apparent when citalopram responders and nonresponders were contrasted, suggesting the potential utility of studying more extreme phenotypes. A subsequent study associated another KCNK2 SNP, rs7549184, with depression severity [6].

A small cohort of individuals with MDD receiving ECT ($n=119$), along with blood donor "controls," have also been studied extensively. Association was reported for a SNP in vascular endothelial growth factor (VEGF) – VEGF2578 [38] – as well as one in tryptophan hydroxylase 1 (TPH1) [41]. (As noted below, the same authors also investigated other candidates including the serotonin 2A receptor (HTR2A) [39], tryptophan hydroxylase 2 (TPH2) [3], and multiple other genes (ACE, RGS4, GNB3).

In a distinct cohort of 190 individuals with MDD, a SNP in CREB1 (rs7569963) was associated with treatment-resistant depression [32]. A subsequent study in 285 individuals with MDD failed to identify association between four other SNPs in CREB1 and TRD, however [4].

In addition to these cohorts of European descent, TRD has been investigated in association studies in Asian populations. In particular, a 2013 multicenter study examined 948 Han Chinese individuals with MDD, including 304 individuals with prospectively established TRD [21]. That study found an association between rs1565445 in neurotrophic tyrosine kinase receptor 2 (NTRK2), the receptor for brain-derived neurotrophic factor, and TRD. Another study in this cohort examined tag SNPs in B-cell lymphoma-2 (BCL2) and found an association between rs2279115 and TRD solely in male subjects [45]. And, yet another study in this cohort identified association with the 2B subunit of the NMDA receptor (GRIN2B) at rs1805502 [44]. (Notably, however, these studies did not control for the multiple genes tested.)

The number of published positive studies unfortunately far exceeds negative studies, suggesting substantial risk of publication bias. Among the negative studies are a recent cohort of 613 MDD patients, including 389 with TRD, where no association was observed with functional SNPs in catechol-O-methyltransferase (COMT) and methylenetetrahydrofolate reductase (MTHFR) [12]. Another investigation of 372 individuals, including a subset with TRD, also did not identify associations with COX2 and OXTR variants [22].

4.4 Treatment Outcomes in TRD Cohorts

While not strictly speaking investigations of TRD risk, other association studies bear consideration as they have investigated response to common treatment options for TRD. Among a cohort of 104 individuals receiving electroconvulsive therapy, multiple SNPs in the dopamine receptor 3 (DRD3) gene were investigated for association with treatment response, and three of these (rs3732790, rs3773679, and rs9817063) were associated with outcome [8]. An interesting feature of this study was inclusion of fMRI with a facial expression paradigm, where the allele associated with better response (rs3732790) also associated with greater striatal responsiveness to happy facial expressions.

Other ECT cohorts have also been investigated for treatment response. In one report, one SNP (rs11030101) in brain-derived neurotrophic factor (BDNF) was associated with response [40]. However, this result must be interpreted in the context of numerous negative associations drawn from the same cohort, including TPH2 [3], angiotensin converting enzyme (ACE) [34], regulator of G protein signaling 4 (RGS4) [18], and apolipoprotein E (APOE) [19]. Another study failed to identify main effects for SNPs in HTR2A previously associated with antidepressant response, although SNP-by-sex effects were suggested [39].

Finally, one study examined response to next-step treatment following SSRI nonresponse with a combination of SNPs across multiple monoaminergic receptors and transporters as well as melanocortin receptors. Among 205 individuals randomized to a combination of olanzapine and fluoxetine, or fluoxetine or olanzapine alone, SNPs in the norepinephrine transporter (SLC6A2), melanocortin receptor 3 (MC3R), and TPH2 were nominally associated with the olanzapine-fluoxetine combination; only the last (TPH2) was also associated with response to the individual treatments [17].

4.5 Clinical Status

To date, none of the results summarized above have been shown to be robust and replicable. On the other hand, multiple medications commonly used to manage TRD have US Food and Drug Administration labeling reflecting genetic data [2]. The majority of these labels relate to variations in the genes coding for the enzymes of the cytochrome p450 system. This palette of enzymes is responsible for hepatic phase I metabolism of many psychotropic medications [see Chap. [3]].

One obvious hypothesis suggests that TRD populations might be enriched for individuals with non-wild-type forms of CYP450 enzymes, in whom effective antidepressant doses would be more difficult to achieve. In particular, individuals with variants conferring ultrarapid metabolism – i.e., greater than typical ability to metabolize particular medications – might be unable to achieve therapeutic antidepressant levels at standard doses. Conversely, those with variants conferring poorer than typical metabolism might be intolerant of antidepressants even at low doses.

Remarkably, only one published study appears to have investigated this question directly [14], among 55 Hungarian patients with TRD. Prevalence of ultrarapid metabolizers was no different from population averages (1.8 % versus 1.9 %); while poor metabolizers were numerically greater (14.5 % versus 8.3 %), the difference was not statistically significant in this very small cohort. (For discussion of the mixed evidence association CYP450 variation with antidepressant response in general, see Chap. [3].)

While cost-effectiveness studies of antidepressant response in general have begun to emerge, the utility of testing treatment-resistant populations in particular has not yet been assessed. The potential value for patients has been addressed in one intriguing Danish survey: patients reported that they would pay approximately $100 to shorten by 1 month the period of antidepressant dose adjustment and $280 to eliminate a single change in medication [16].

4.6 Challenges and Future Directions

A major challenge in studying the biological basis of treatment resistance in major depressive disorder is excluding what has been referred to as pseudoresistance (Table 4.1): individuals whose poor response to medications is driven by nonadherence, inadequate dosing or duration, and/or adverse events. Nonadherence in particular may impact up to half the participants in the sorts of clinical investigations often used to derive pharmacogenomics cohorts [5, 33, 42]. Of course, many of these factors may themselves be influenced by genetic variation – for example, cytochrome p450 variations causing patients to develop abnormally high serum levels even with low doses, yielding adverse effects that contribute to nonadherence. Still, distinguishing true treatment resistance (i.e., inability to respond despite adequate treatment trials) from these other factors may be difficult without longitudinal assessment. Moreover, a commonly overlooked problem is the extent to which efficacy may be confounded by adverse effects or vice versa. (See, e.g., Keers [20].)

Table 4.1 Key considerations in pharmacogenomic studies of treatment-resistant depression	
	Medication adherence
	Adverse effects/intolerance
	Adequate treatment duration
	Outcome definition (improvement/response/remission)
	Inclusion of non-antidepressant concomitant treatments
	Phenocopies/medical comorbidity
	Comparison groups for TRD cohort

Table 4.2 Study designs for TRD

Source	Outcome data	Treatment data	Randomization	DNA	Sample size	Relative cost
Clinical trial	+++	+++	Yes	+++	+	$$$
Cohort study or disease registry	++	++	No	+++	+/++	$$
Health claims data	+	+	No	Requires recontact	+++	$
Electronic health record	++	++	No	Requires recontact or biobank	+++	$

That is, patients may be more likely to continue a treatment in spite of limited tolerability if they perceive benefit from it. As such, strategies which claim to distinguish efficacy from tolerability may be somewhat naïve – it is the rare antidepressant treatment-adherent patient who experiences/no/adverse effects, however mild.

A related problem is the range of medical comorbidities that may contribute either to persistence of MDD or to depressive symptoms. Two examples are hypothyroidism (regardless of etiology) and sleep apnea, both of which may contribute to apparent treatment resistance. While the importance of these factors in unselected clinical populations is difficult to estimate, unless specifically excluded, they may contribute heterogeneity to the population of patients with TRD. (As with adverse effects, these factors may themselves be genetic, of course.)

While these TRD phenocopies undoubtedly contribute to misclassification and thus diminish the power of association studies to identify risk variants, the greatest limitation in such studies remains the paucity of samples available for study. Indeed, across psychiatric genomics, after decades of argument about correctness of phenotypes and other strategies required for success, efforts to identify common genetic association have begun to succeed largely because of adequately powered sample cohorts combined via meta-analysis. As with antidepressant response genomics as a whole [30], it is fair to say such sample sizes have not yet been achieved in the study of treatment-resistant depression.

As such, a key next step in the study of treatment resistance is achieving such cohorts. (While the precise sample size needed for success in genome-wide study varies widely, nearly all phenotypes have yielded to cohorts of 10,000 cases or more.) Of course, if this process has proven challenging for disease phenotypes, collecting cohorts requiring establishment of diagnosis plus two (or more) treatment trials is likely to be substantially more so.

There are at least three possible next steps, and all of these may be required in order to find reliable, replicable associations. First, investigators will likely need to share data in the context of a consortium. Second, the largely untapped data from large randomized trials conducted by pharmaceutical companies will need to become accessible. And finally, novel means of identifying cases and controls from large-scale biobanks, registries, or repositories may be required to augment the data available from costly prospective clinical trials (Table 4.2). An example of such an initiative was the rare variant study of TRD described earlier, in which treatment response was characterized based on electronic health records [28]. This approach may also facilitate the development of integrated risk models incorporating both genetic and clinical risk predictors [27].

TRD remains an area of great clinical importance in psychiatry, contributing substantially to morbidity and healthcare cost. The lack of success in identifying reliable risk variants to date likely reflects a problem of engineering, not science: investigators will need to collect sufficiently large cohorts to afford adequate statistical power. In light of the potential benefit that early identification of TRD risk could afford, however, further efforts to efficiently characterize such cohorts are sorely needed.

References

1. Alexanderson B, Evans DA, Sjoqvist F (1969) Steady-state plasma levels of nortriptyline in twins: influence of genetic factors and drug therapy. Br Med J 4(5686):764–768
2. Anonymous (2014) Table of pharmacogenomic biomarkers in drug labeling, [online]. Available: http://www.fda.gov/drugs/scienceresearch/researchareas/pharmacogenetics/ucm083378.htm
3. Anttila S, Viikki M, Huuhka K, Huuhka M, Huhtala H, Rontu R et al (2009) TPH2 polymorphisms may modify clinical picture in treatment-resistant depression. Neurosci Lett 464(1): 43–46
4. Calati R, Crisafulli C, Balestri M, Serretti A, Spina E, Calabrò M et al (2013) Evaluation of the role of MAPK1 and CREB1 polymorphisms on treatment resistance, response and remission in mood disorder patients. Prog Neuropsychopharmacol Biol Psychiatry 44:271–278
5. Cantrell CR, Eaddy MT, Shah MB, Regan TS, Sokol MC (2006) Methods for evaluating patient adherence to antidepressant therapy: a real-world comparison of adherence and economic outcomes. Med Care 44(4):300–303
6. Congiu C, Minelli A, Bonvicini C, Bortolomasi M, Sartori R, Maj C et al (2015) The role of the potassium channel gene KCNK2 in major depressive disorder. Psychiatry Res 225(3): 489–492
7. Crowley JJ, Brodkin ES, Blendy JA, Berrettini WH, Lucki I (2006) Pharmacogenomic evaluation of the antidepressant citalopram in the mouse tail suspension test. Neuropsychopharmacology 31(11):2433–2442
8. Dannlowski U, Domschke K, Birosova E, Lawford B, Young R, Voisey J et al (2013) Dopamine D3 receptor gene variation: impact on electroconvulsive therapy response and ventral striatum responsiveness in depression. Int J Neuropsychopharmacol 16(7):1443–1459
9. Fava M, Rush AJ, Trivedi MH, Nierenberg AA, Thase ME, Sackeim HA et al (2003) Background and rationale for the sequenced treatment alternatives to relieve depression (STAR*D) study. Psychiatr Clin North Am 26(2):457–494, x
10. Fountoulakis KN, Moller HJ (2011) Efficacy of antidepressants: a re-analysis and re-interpretation of the Kirsch data. Int J Neuropsychopharmacol 14(3):405–412
11. Franchini L, Serretti A, Gasperini M, Smeraldi E (1998) Familial concordance of fluvoxamine response as a tool for differentiating mood disorder pedigrees. J Psychiatr Res 32(5): 255–259
12. Gabriela Nielsen M, Congiu C, Bortolomasi M, Bonvicini C, Bignotti S, Abate M et al (2015) MTHFR: Genetic variants, expression analysis and COMT interaction in major depressive disorder. J Affect Disord 183:179–186
13. Gibson TB, Jing Y, Smith Carls G, Kim E, Bagalman JE, Burton WN et al (2010) Cost burden of treatment resistance in patients with depression. Am J Manag Care 16(5):370–377

14. Háber A, Rideg O, Osváth P, Fekete S, Szücs F, Fittler A et al (2013) Patients with difficult-to-treat depression do not exhibit an increased frequency of CYP2D6 allele duplication. Pharmacopsychiatry 46(4):156–160
15. Heimann H (1974) Therapy-resistant depressions: symptoms and syndromes. Contributions to symptomatology and syndromes. Pharmakopsychiatr Neuropsychopharmakol 7(3):139–144
16. Herbild L, Bech M, Gyrd-Hansen D (2009) Estimating the Danish populations' preferences for pharmacogenetic testing using a discrete choice experiment. The case of treating depression. Value Health 12(4):560–567
17. Houston JP, Lau K, Aris V, Liu W, Fijal BA, Heinloth AN, Perlis RH (2012) Association of common variations in the norepinephrine transporter gene with response to olanzapine-fluoxetine combination versus continued-fluoxetine treatment in patients with treatment-resistant depression: a candidate gene analysis. J Clin Psychiatry 73(6):878–885
18. Huuhka K, Kampman O, Anttila S, Huuhka M, Rontu R, Mattila KM et al (2008) RGS4 polymorphism and response to electroconvulsive therapy in major depressive disorder. Neurosci Lett 437(1):25–28
19. Huuhka M, Anttila S, Leinonen E, Huuhka K, Rontu R, Mattila KM et al (2005) The apolipoprotein E polymorphism is not associated with response to electroconvulsive therapy in major depressive disorder. J ECT 21(1):7–11
20. Keers R, Bonvicini C, Scassellati C, Uher R, Placentino A, Giovannini C et al (2011) Variation in GNB3 predicts response and adverse reactions to antidepressants. J Psychopharmacol 25(7):867–874
21. Li Z, Zhang Y, Wang Z, Chen J, Fan J, Guan Y et al (2013) The role of BDNF, NTRK2 gene and their interaction in development of treatment-resistant depression: data from multicenter, prospective, longitudinal clinic practice. J Psychiatr Res 47(1):8–14
22. Mendlewicz J, Crisafulli C, Calati R, Kocabas NA, Massat I, Linotte S et al (2012) Influence of COX-2 and OXTR polymorphisms on treatment outcome in treatment resistant depression. Neurosci Lett 516(1):85–88
23. O'Reilly RL, Bogue L, Singh SM (1994) Pharmacogenetic response to antidepressants in a multicase family with affective disorder. Biol Psychiatry 36(7):467–471
24. Oquendo MA, Baca-Garcia E, Kartachov A, Khait V, Campbell CE, Richards M et al (2003) A computer algorithm for calculating the adequacy of antidepressant treatment in unipolar and bipolar depression. J Clin Psychiatry 64(7):825–833
25. Pare CM, Rees L, Sainsbury MJ (1962) Differentiation of two genetically specific types of depression by the response to anti-depressants. Lancet 2(7270):1340–1343
26. Perlis R (2014) Pharmacogenomic testing and personalized treatment of depression. Clin Chem 60(1):53–59
27. Perlis RH (2013) A clinical risk stratification tool for predicting treatment resistance in major depressive disorder. Biol Psychiatry 74(1):7–14
28. Perlis RH, Iosifescu DV, Castro V, Murphy S, Gainer V, Minnier J et al (2012) Using electronic medical records to enable large-scale studies in psychiatry: treatment resistant depression as a model. Psychol Med 42(1):41–50
29. Perlis RH, Moorjani P, Fagerness J, Purcell S, Trivedi MH, Fava M et al (2008) Pharmacogenetic analysis of genes implicated in rodent models of antidepressant response: association of TREK1 and treatment resistance in the STAR(*)D study. Neuropsychopharmacology 33(12):2810–2819
30. Ripke S, O'Dushlaine C, Chambert K, Moran JL, Kahler AK, Akterin S et al (2013) Genome-wide association analysis identifies 13 new risk loci for schizophrenia. Nat Genet 45(10):1150–9
31. Rush A, Trivedi M, Wisniewski S, Nierenberg A, Stewart J, Warden D et al (2006) Acute and longer-term outcomes in depressed outpatients requiring one or several treatment steps: a STAR*D report. Am J Psychiatry 163(11):1905–1917
32. Serretti A, Chiesa A, Calati R, Massat I, Linotte S, Kasper S et al (2011) A preliminary investigation of the influence of CREB1 gene on treatment resistance in major depression. J Affect Disord 128(1–2):56–63

33. Stein MB, Cantrell CR, Sokol MC, Eaddy MT, Shah MB (2006) Antidepressant adherence and medical resource use among managed care patients with anxiety disorders. Psychiatr Serv 57(5):673–680
34. Stewart JA, Kampman O, Huuhka M, Anttila S, Huuhka K, Lehtimäki T et al (2009) ACE polymorphism and response to electroconvulsive therapy in major depression. Neurosci Lett 458(3):122–125
35. Tansey KE, Guipponi M, Hu X, Domenici E, Lewis G, Malafosse A et al (2013) Contribution of common genetic variants to antidepressant response. Biol Psychiatry 73(7):679–682
36. Tansey KE, Rucker JJ, Kavanagh DH, Guipponi M, Perroud N, Bondolfi G et al (2014) Copy number variants and therapeutic response to antidepressant medication in major depressive disorder. Pharmacogenomics J 14(4):395–399
37. Thase ME, Rush AJ (1997) When at first you don't succeed: sequential strategies for antidepressant nonresponders. J Clin Psychiatry 59(Suppl(13)):23–29
38. Viikki M, Anttila S, Kampman O, Illi A, Huuhka M, Setälä-Soikkeli E et al (2010) Vascular endothelial growth factor (VEGF) polymorphism is associated with treatment resistant depression. Neurosci Lett 477(3):105–108
39. Viikki M, Huuhka K, Leinonen E, Illi A, Setälä-Soikkeli E, Huuhka M et al (2011) Interaction between two HTR2A polymorphisms and gender is associated with treatment response in MDD. Neurosci Lett 501(1):20–24
40. Viikki M, Jarventausta K, Leinonen E, Huuhka K, Mononen N, Lehtimäki T, Kampman O (2013) BDNF polymorphism rs11030101 is associated with the efficacy of electroconvulsive therapy in treatment-resistant depression. Psychiatr Genet 23(3):134–136
41. Viikki M, Kampman O, Illi A, Setälä-Soikkeli E, Anttila S, Huuhka M et al (2010) TPH1 218A/C polymorphism is associated with major depressive disorder and its treatment response. Neurosci Lett 468(1):80–84
42. Warden D, Trivedi MH, Carmody T, Toups M, Zisook S, Lesser I et al (2014) Adherence to antidepressant combinations and monotherapy for major depressive disorder: a CO-MED report of measurement-based care. J Psychiatr Pract 20(2):118–132
43. Zarate C, Duman RS, Liu G, Sartori S, Quiroz J, Murck H (2013) New paradigms for treatment-resistant depression. Ann N Y Acad Sci 1292:21–31
44. Zhang C, Li Z, Wu Z, Chen J, Wang Z, Peng D et al (2014) A study of N-methyl-D-aspartate receptor gene (GRIN2B) variants as predictors of treatment-resistant major depression. Psychopharmacology (Berl) 231(4):685–693
45. Zhang L, Evans DS, Raheja UK, Stephens SH, Stiller JW, Reeves GM et al (2015) Chronotype and seasonality: morningness is associated with lower seasonal mood and behavior changes in the Old Order Amish. J Affect Disord 174:209–214

Chapter 5
Complementation of Pharmacogenetics with Biomarkers and Neuroimaging in Major Depression

Andreas Menke, Nicola Dusi, and Paolo Brambilla

Abstract Unlike other disciplines of medicine, the diagnostic process in psychiatry is based solely on clinical judgment, without incorporating lab-derived objective measures on a regular basis. Even with the advent of DMS-V, no biomarkers gathered from genomics, peripheral blood, or brain imaging have been established for the diagnostic process in psychiatric disorders. However, there is accumulating evidence of evolving biomarkers to improve diagnostic processes and treatment algorithm. Here, studies on the evaluation of markers derived from imaging and peripheral blood in patients with major depression are reviewed. An altered brain network that encompasses the anterior cingulate, the prefrontal cortex, and the hippocampus has been repeatedly found in major depression. Antidepressants exert neuroprotective effects, which determine a reduction of hippocampal and prefrontal cortex shrinkage, probably through an activation of neuromodulatory factors like BDNF. Lower BDNF plasma levels are observed in depressed patients and normalize after successful treatment. Very promising findings have also been observed within inflammatory pathways and the hypothalamic–pituitary–adrenal (HPA) axis. In both systems, there is growing evidence that drugs specifically targeting these

A. Menke (✉)
Department of Psychiatry, Psychosomatics and Psychotherapy,
University Hospital of Würzburg, Würzburg, Germany
e-mail: Menke_A@ukw.de

N. Dusi
Section of Psychiatry, Department of Public Health and Community Medicine,
Inter-University Center for Behavioral Neurosciences (ICBN), University of Verona,
Verona, Italy

P. Brambilla
Department of Neurosciences and Mental Health,
Fondazione IRCCS Ca' Granda Ospedale Maggiore Policlinico,
University of Milan, Milan, Italy

Scientific Institute IRCCS "E. Medea", Bosisio Parini (Lc), Italy

Department of Psychiatry and Behavioral Sciences,
University of Texas Health Science Center at Houston, TX, USA

© Springer International Publishing Switzerland 2016
J.K. Rybakowski, A. Serretti (eds.), *Genetic Influences on Response to Drug Treatment for Major Psychiatric Disorders*, DOI 10.1007/978-3-319-27040-1_5

systems may be beneficial for the treatment of depression, but only in these patients, who have marked alterations detected by the respective biomarkers.

5.1 Introduction

In the last 30 years, there has been an increasing interest on the research for neuro-biological underpinnings of psychiatric disorders, since they represent a growing and worrying cause of disability and poor quality of life worldwide, but little is still understood about their etiology, the mechanisms behind the development of this wide family of disorders, and their treatment [25, 88]. Diagnoses in psychiatry are still based on syndromic descriptions, which have a large range of manifestations and severity, and rely on symptoms that often overlap between disorders. One strategy to overcome the heterogeneity of psychiatric diagnoses would be the identification of more homogenous groups of patients, who share similar clinical features and, possibly, more similar endophenotypes. This approach would help biological research in the discovery of putative alterations of brain disorders and clinical practice in the applications of specific tailored strategies of intervention on narrower patients' populations [8]. In this perspective, structural magnetic resonance can be a useful tool in the research of markers of treatment response and clinical course in major psychiatric disorders [7].

Another approach to foster personalized medicine is the investigation of blood-based biomarkers. Peripheral blood represents an attractive tissue source since it is easily accessible for single diagnostic assessments or for continuous monitoring surveillance. While peripheral blood cells are not likely to reflect signatures in neuronal cells, they are in contact with every tissue in the body, including the brain, and, for example, studies on gene expression observed 82 % co-expressed genes in human peripheral blood and brain tissue [61]. In addition, the retrieval and analyses of blood is not an expensive approach.

This chapter will focus on the main hypotheses of altered systems, inflammation, the hypothalamic–pituitary–adrenal axis, and neuronal plasticity, along with structural imaging features of illness severity and treatment response, in mood disorders, particularly depressive disorder.

5.2 Blood-Based Biomarkers

5.2.1 Inflammation

Accumulating evidence suggests that inflammation plays a subtle role in the patho-physiology in mood disorders. There are three major observations linking inflammation to major depression: patients with major depression show elevated peripheral inflammatory markers, even in the absence of a systemic infection; inflammatory diseases are associated with increased rates to develop major depression; and patients treated with cytokines like interferon-α (IFN-α) and IL-2 are at greater risk for a depressive episode. Confirmed by two recent meta-analyses, the most replicated findings of increased inflammatory markers in serum or CSF collected from depressed patients pertain C-reactive protein (CRP, a commonly marker of systemic inflammation), TNF-α, and IL-6 [62]. In addition, a meta-analysis of 22 antidepressant treatment studies found a decrease of IL-1β and IL-6 levels in patients successfully responding to treatment. Interestingly, in a meta-analysis on blood-borne biomarkers predicting mortality risk the two with inflammatory processes-associated markers, CRP and white blood cell count, showed the highest association with mortality risk among the investigated 51 blood-borne biomarkers [4].

Based on the hypothesis of an exaggeration of inflammatory processes in mood disorders, an en bloc assessment of a set of biomarkers covering the three dimensions neurotrophins (brain-derived neurotrophic factor, neurotrophin-3), oxidative stress markers (protein carbonyl content, thiobarbituric acid reactive substances, total reactive antioxidant potentials), and inflammatory markers (interleukin-6, interleukin-10, and tumor necrosis factor α) was studied in a sample of euthymic, manic, and depressed bipolar patients as well as healthy controls and patients suffering from sepsis [50]. This set of biomarkers was regarded as a proxy of systemic toxicity and termed the systemic toxicity index (STI). While there were no differences between healthy controls and euthymic bipolar patients, depressed as well as manic patients exhibited a significant increased STI. Patients with sepsis showed the highest values of the STI. This study described a substantial increment of inflammatory processes in bipolar disorder, interestingly similar for manic and depressed patients, pointing out a toxicity against multiple cellular elements in the body [50].

5.2.1.1 Predicting Treatment Response

Several studies explored the usefulness of inflammatory markers to predict treatment response in major depression. Increased levels of IL-6 were found in patients failing response to SSRI or amitriptyline treatment, and raised TNF-α levels were found in SSRI nonresponders. Harley et al. showed that patients with CRP baseline levels above 10 mg/l responded better to therapy with nortriptyline or fluoxetine than to psychotherapy (interpersonal therapy, IPT or CBT) [38]. This very interesting finding for treatment stratification is somewhat compromised by the study design. Two independently recruited samples were analyzed with one sample comparing patients treated with fluoxetine and nortriptyline and one sample randomizing patients to IPT and CBT. Next, patients in the medication study being nonresponsive to the drug were switched to the other antidepressant; hence, there is no information on the specific response rate of the antidepressants in relation to CRP levels [38].

However, another study observed beneficial effects of nortriptyline after stratifying for CRP levels. CRP was tested as a predictor for treatment response in a cohort of 241 depressed participants of the Genome-Based Therapeutic Drugs for Depression (GENDEP) study, a multicenter open-label randomized clinical trial [98]. Patients were randomly allocated to 12-week treatment with escitalopram or nortriptyline. Interestingly, CRP levels at baseline differentially predicted treatment outcome. For patients with low CRP levels (<1 mg/l), improvement on the MADRS score was 3 points higher with escitalopram than with nortriptyline. Contrary, patients with higher CRP levels exhibited 3 points greater improvement on the MADRS score with nortriptyline than with escitalopram [98]. This would be an easily accessible peripheral blood biomarker; replication in a larger sample would accentuate its relevance. Different effects of selective reuptake inhibitors and tricyclic antidepressants on immune cells or associated factors were also observed in vitro. In blood cultures of healthy female subjects, tricyclic antidepressants significantly suppressed interferon-gamma (IFN-gamma) concentrations, while there were no significant effects of the SNRI venlafaxine [42].

These findings foster the hypothesis that anti-inflammatory medication would be a treatment option in depression or at least an improvement of established therapies. Studies observed already a beneficial effect of anti-inflammatory medication as add-on to antidepressant medication [71] and as monotherapy [46]; however, an analysis of data from the Sequenced Treatment Alternative to Relieve Depression (STAR*D) indicated that anti-inflammatory drugs may also have antagonistic effects on the effectiveness of SSRIs [103]. A recent meta-analysis including 14 trials evaluating the use of nonsteroidal anti-inflammatory drugs (NSAIDs) and cytokine inhibitors in 6262 participants suggested an improvement of depressive symptoms without increased risks of adverse effects [53]. Of note, one study enrolling 60 depressed patients who were subject to either infusion with the TNF antagonist infliximab or placebo revealed no overall difference between the treatment groups [82]. However, there was a significant interaction between treatment type and baseline CRP levels, favoring infliximab-treated patients at a baseline CRP concentration greater than 5 mg/L [82]. In a further exploration of response predictors, mRNA profiles derived from peripheral blood mononuclear cells from infliximab responders (n=13) vs. nonresponders (n=14) were compared. One hundred forty-eight transcripts were significantly associated with response to infliximab and were distinct from placebo response. Transcripts belonged to gluconeogenesis and cholesterol transport pathways.

5.2.2 HPA Axis

A dysregulation of the hypothalamic–pituitary–adrenal (HPA) axis in patients suffering from major depression has been robustly demonstrated [43]. The negative feedback mechanisms, usually controlling peripheral cortisol levels, are in depressed patients impaired, and thus the secretion of corticotropin-releasing hormone (CRH) is increased which results in an enhanced ACTH and subsequently cortisol production [43]. There are two common endocrine tests, which are usually applied to examine the HPA axis in psychiatric disorders, the dexamethasone-suppression test (DST) [15] and the dexamethasone–corticotropin-releasing hormone (dex-CRH) test [41]. The dexamethasone-suppression test, in which an escape from the suppressive effect of dexamethasone on cortisol has been observed in depressed patient, has been initially described in the 1970s [15]. Although there were several supportive findings for the utility of the DST to identify patients with depression [72] and predict clinical outcome, widespread use of the DST as a diagnostic tool was limited by the tests of low sensitivity, ranging between 20 and 50 % [74]. To develop a more sensitive test detecting HPA axis dysregulation, the DST was combined with the CRH stimulation test; this appeared to improve sensitivity to over 80 % to detect an HPA dysregulation and identify depressed patients [41]. While these initial findings could be replicated by some studies [45, 57, 92], there were other studies reporting inconsistent results when analyzing case/control differences [14]. In addition to possible case identification, several reports suggest that the dex-CRH test may allow substratification of patients with depression. Several studies observed an exaggerated ACTH and cortisol response to the dex-CRH test in remitted patients subject to clinical relapse [3, 45], in melancholic patients compared to non-melancholic depressed patients [49], and in individuals with violent suicide attempts and ultimately suicide completion [23]. In contrast, significantly attenuated cortisol and ACTH responses in the dex-CRH test were observed in depressed women with chronic social stressors [85] and in depressed patients with suicidal behavior [79]. A study by Paslakis et al. compared diurnal (24 h) cortisol profiles with DST and dex-CRH test outcomes to discriminate depressed patients and healthy controls. Diurnal cortisol profiles outperformed DST and dex-CRH test outcomes, with an optimal time interval between 10:00 and 12:00 h with a sensitivity of 83 % and specificity of 87 %. However, this study reanalyzed previously collected data and included only 26 patients and 33 controls [77].

Next to the measurement of peripheral cortisol and ACTH, the glucocorticoid receptor (GR) itself is an interesting target, as it plays an important role in mediating the negative feedback regulation of the HPA axis [34]. Two isoforms of the GR have been described, GRα and GRβ, which have distinct biological activity. Matsubara et al. found a significantly reduced GRα mRNA expression in peripheral blood cells of depressed patients compared to healthy controls [65]. Interestingly, even patients already remitted from major depression showed reduced GRα mRNA expression [65].

A crucial mediator of the HPA axis is the FK506-binding protein 51, or FKBP5, a cochaperone of the heat shock protein 90 [10]. FKBP5 is supposed to regulate GR sensitivity: when it is bound to the receptor complex of the GR, cortisol binds with lower affinity, and nuclear translocation of the receptor is less efficient [10]. The group of Elisabeth Binder at the Max Planck Institute of Psychiatry in Munich studied GR-induced gene expression profiles in whole blood in vivo [68]. Dexamethasone was orally administered to depressed patients and healthy controls. After dexamethasone stimulation, the number and the extent of the regulated transcripts favored a reduced GR sensitivity in depressed patients compared to healthy controls. FKBP5 mRNA was one of the top regulated genes; depressed patients displayed a significantly reduced FKBP5 mRNA expression due to dexamethasone intake [68]. A further study investigating GR-stimulated FKBP5 mRNA expression in whole blood of patients suffering from major depression observed a significant attenuated FKBP5 mRNA induction after dexamethasone intake only in patients carrying the risk allele of the rs1360780 FKBP5 polymorphism [69]. This was paralleled by the extent of plasma cortisol and ACTH suppression, with a reduced suppression only found in depressed patients carrying the risk allele. The same approach to study GR sensitivity was applied in subjects suffering from job-related exhaustion. Dexamethasone-induced gene expression indicated a GR hypersensitivity, which was normalized after 12 weeks of standardized aerobic exercise [67]. Since these studies were conducted only with small sample sizes, the results await further replication to strengthen the validity of this molecular dexamethasone test to assess GR functioning.

Altered FKBP5 mRNA levels were also found in the Genome-Based Therapeutic Drugs for Depression (GENDEP) project, a multicenter pharmacogenetic study with depressed patients treated with either escitalopram or nortriptyline [97]. Following a successful antidepressant treatment, a significant reduction of FKBP5 mRNA levels in peripheral blood was observed [17]. Katz et al. investigated the mRNA expression of genes involved in GR signaling in whole blood of women with a history of mood disorders from preconception through the third trimester of pregnancy and observed an upregulation of GR complex-regulating genes over pregnancy [51]. Interestingly, in women with depressive symptoms, the increase in expression of FKBP5, BCL2-associated athanogene (BAG1), nuclear receptor coactivator 1 (NCOA1), and peptidylprolyl isomerase D (PPID) was significantly smaller. Ex vivo stimulation assays showed that GR sensitivity was diminished with progression of pregnancy and increasing maternal depressive symptoms [51]. If replicated, the peripheral expression of GR cochaperone genes may serve as biomarkers for the risk of developing depressive symptoms during pregnancy.

The retinoid-related orphan receptor alpha (RORa) has recently gained attention as a new candidate in stress-related diseases, especially depression. The transcription factor RORa is a clock gene which belongs to the steroid hormone receptor superfamily and was associated with the response to cellular stress [47]. There is some evidence suggesting that an altered molecular clock is involved in the pathophysiology of depression. A study analyzed genome-wide transcripts in peripheral blood of 12 remitters, and 12 nonresponders to antidepressant treatment found a lower expression of retinoid-related orphan receptor alpha (RORa), germinal center-expressed transcript 2 (GCET2), and chitinase 3-like protein 2 (CHI3L2) on admission in participant remitting patients. Peripheral blood was obtained at admission after 2 and 5 weeks. Successful replication was achieved in an independent sample of 142 depressed patients [40].

5.2.2.1 Treatment Implications

Based on the hypothesis of a dysregulated HPA axis in patients with psychotic depression, a treatment with mifepristone, which is not only an antiprogesterone but also at high concentrations, a GR antagonist in vitro and in vivo was investigated. In small samples, mifepristone could actually attenuate depressive symptoms significantly better than placebo treatment [6, 27]. However, a recent meta-analysis over studies investigating antiglucocorticoid treatments for unipolar or bipolar depression, including mifepristone, ketoconazole, metyrapone, or dehydroepiandrosterone (DHEA), did not reveal substantial beneficial effects in the treatment of depression [33]. However, there were large methodological differences between studies with respect to the compounds used and patient cohort studies. Particularly, it was noted that the findings in some diagnostic subtypes were promising and warrant further investigation to establish the clinical utility of these drugs in the treatment of mood disorders [33].

A very new approach to target the HPA axis is modulating FKBP51. Drug discovery for FKBP51 has been limited by the inability to pharmacologically differentiate against the structurally similar but functional opposing homolog FKBP52, and all known FKBP ligands were unselective [31]. Meanwhile, a new class of ligands could be developed with an induced-fit mechanism selectively targeting FKBP51 [31]. These new substances could already enhance neurite elongation in neuronal cultures and improve neuroendocrine feedback and stress-coping behavior in mice [31].

5.2.3 Adrenergic Nervous System

The adrenergic nervous system (ANS) is another stress system supposed to be dysregulated in psychiatric disorders, especially in major depression. Additionally, the HPA axis and the ANS seem to be connected, for example, a positive correlation of plasma norepinephrine and cortisol has been observed [84]. Cerebrospinal fluid (CSF) levels of the norepinephrine metabolite 3-methoxy-4-hydroxyphenylglycol (MHPG) have been suggested as a biomarker for suicide risk [32]. For example, a prospective study analyzed the relationship between MHPG levels and suicidal behavior in 184 subjects with unipolar and bipolar depression. Lower concentrations of the norepinephrine metabolite were predictive of suicidal behavior and were correlated with higher medical lethality of the future suicide attempt [32]. Also norepinephrine itself was implicated with depression. A study comparing depressive symptoms between caregivers and non-caregivers revealed a prolonged activated plasma norepinephrine response following a laboratory-based stress paradigm in depressed caregivers [2].

5.2.4 Neural Plasticity

There is accumulating evidence for a reduced neuronal plasticity in various psychiatric disorders. The brain-derived neurotrophic factor BDNF belongs to the neurotrophins, which modulate migration, proliferation, and differentiation of neurons in the human central nervous system. Additionally, BDNF was associated with treatment response to antidepressants and antipsychotics [70]. As BDNF crosses the blood-brain barrier, and shows a high correlation of its levels in CSF and serum, it is regarded as a "window to the brain" and thus enables it as a suitable biomarker for neuropsychiatric disorders.

BDNF RNA expression in peripheral lymphocytes was decreased in depressed patients compared to healthy controls [75]. An increase in BDNF and VGF nerve growth factor RNA expression was observed in depressed patients responding to treatment with escitalopram or nortriptyline within the GENDEP project [18]. The increase of BDNF RNA expression following successful therapy with antidepressants was paralleled by BDNF serum increase which also correlated with an improvement of symptoms [16]. In addition, VGF RNA expression derived from peripheral leucocytes of medication-free depressed patients was significantly reduced before treatment and was modulated in response to effective antidepressant treatment [18].

A comparative meta-analysis of studies investigating BDNF serum and plasma levels in patients suffering from MDD, bipolar disorder, and schizophrenia revealed strong effect sizes of BDNF to discriminate healthy controls or remitted patients with mood disorders against mood disorder patients in an acute episode or patients with schizophrenia. However, BDNF levels could not distinguish between remitted patients and healthy controls or between depressed, manic, and schizophrenic patients [26].

The vascular endothelial growth factor (VEGF) has been implicated in neurotrophic models of depression. A study found significantly increased plasma VEGF levels in depressed patients compared to healthy controls. A 63 % overall discrimination between depressed and healthy participants could be achieved by analyzing plasma VEGF levels [20]. A study investigating 34 depressed patients found a trend of higher plasma VEGF levels in nonresponders compared to responders to antidepressant treatment at baseline [37].

Xiong et al. compared protein levels derived from the sera of 278 schizophrenia patients, 240 depression and bipolar patients, and 260 healthy controls. They found significantly lower serum BDNF, MBP, and GFAP levels and higher serum IL-6 and S100b levels in schizophrenic patients [104]. Applying receiver-operating characteristic (ROC), curve analysis delivered a significant discrimination between schizophrenic patients and controls (AUC=0.922) and the depression and bipolar participants (AUC=0.762).

Table 15.1 Structural magnetic resonance studies on volumetric brain effects of antidepressants

Author	Subjects	Treatment	Brain areas	Results
Vakili et al. [100]	38 patients (17 males, mean age 38.5 ± 10.0 years) 20 healthy controls (9 males, mean age 40.3 ± 10.4 years)	Fluoxetine, 20 mg/day Prospective, 8 weeks	Hippocampus	Larger right hippocampal volume in female responders vs. nonresponders
Salloway et al. (2002) [86]	59 patients under sertraline (mean age 69.22 ± 5.63 years) 111 patients under citalopram (mean age 79.43 ± 4.13 years)	Sertraline, citalopram Prospective, 8 weeks Open label	Subcortical hyperintensities	Larger level of subcortical hyperintensities in citalopram group vs. sertraline group, strong correlation with age No correlation between subcortical hyperintensities and treatment response
Hsieh et al. [44]	60 patients (24 males, mean age 68.57 ± 6.43 years)	Multiple treatment (SSRIs, bupropion, venlafaxine, nefazodone, mirtazapine, nortriptyline) Prospective, 12 weeks	Hippocampus	Smaller right hippocampal volume in nonremitting patients vs. remitting patients
Pizzagalli et al. [81]	20 melancholic patients (7 males, mean age 36.57 ± 12.9 years) 18 non-melancholic patients (8 males, mean age 33.17 ± 8.8 years) 18 healthy controls (8 males, mean age 38.1 ± 13.6 years)	Nortriptyline up to 150 ng/ml Longitudinal, 6 months	Automated analysis	No volumetric differences between groups
Frodl et al. [28]	30 patients (12 males, mean age 48,4 ± 13,9 years) 30 healthy controls (12 males, mean age 45,7 ± 12,9 years)	Multiple drugs (fluvoxamine, paroxetine, sertraline, citalopram, venlafaxine, mirtazapine, amitriptyline, doxepin, trimipramine, and reboxetine) Longitudinal, 1 year f-up	Amygdala, hippocampus	Smaller bilateral hippocampal volumes in nonremitting patients vs. remitted patients, both at baseline and at f-up

(continued)

Table 15.1 (continued)

Author	Subjects	Treatment	Brain areas	Results
Vythilingam et al. [102]	38 patients (15 males, mean age 41 ± 11 years) 33 healthy controls (12 males, mean age 34 ± 10 years)	Multiple drugs *Longitudinal: remission (22 patients, 20 fluoxetine, 1 venlafaxine, 1 sertraline) (subanalysis with 20 patients: fluoxetine)* Longitudinal, 7 ± 3 months	Hippocampus and temporal lobe	No treatment effect
Lavretsky et al. [59]	11 treatment exposure patients (4 males, mean age 67 ± 6.1 years) 30 drug-naive patients (5 males, mean age 71.7 ± 7.8 years) 41 healthy controls (21 males, mean age 72.2 ± 7.3 years)	Multiple drugs Cross-sectional	Automated analysis	Larger OFC GM volumes in treated depressed patients compared to drug-naive depressed patients, but smaller than those in normal controls
Papakostas et al. [77]	50 patients (33 males, mean age 41.2 ± 10.2 years)	Fluoxetine, 20 mg/day Prospective, 8 weeks	Subcortical and periventricular WM hyperintensities	Greater severity of hyperintensities in nonresponders vs. responders
Chen et al. [19]	17 patients (5 males, mean age 44.06 ± 8.36 years)	Fluoxetine, 20 mg/day Prospective, 8 weeks	Automated analysis	Larger GM volume in anterior cingulate cortex, insula, and right temporoparietal cortex in responders vs. nonresponders
Colla et al. [22]	24 patients (9 males, mean age 54.5 ± 11.9 years) 14 healthy controls (6 males, mean age 53.8 ± 17.7 years)	Paroxetine, up to 40 mg/day Amitriptyline, up to 150 mg/day Prospective, 4 weeks	Hippocampus	No treatment effect

		Automated analysis	F-up:
Frodl et al. [28][a]	38 patients (13 males, mean age 46.1±11.3 years) 30 healthy controls (11 males, mean age 43.6±11.3 years)	Multiple drugs (*fluvoxamine, paroxetine, sertraline, citalopram, venlafaxine, mirtazapine, amitriptyline, doxepin, trimipramine, and reboxetine*) Longitudinal, 3 years f-up	Smaller decline in left hippocampus, left anterior cingulum, left dorsomedial prefrontal cortex, and bilateral dorsolateral prefrontal cortex in remitting patients vs. nonremitting
MacQueen et al. [64]	14 remitted patients (8 males, mean age 30.5±9.5 years) 32 nonremitted patients (15 males, mean age 27.6±10.5 years)	Multiple drugs (*citalopram, venlafaxine, bupropion, mirtazapine, sertraline, and fluvoxamine*) Prospective, 8 weeks	Hippocampus — Larger pretreatment hippocampal body/tail volume in remitted patients vs. nonremitted patients
Kronmüller et al. [56]	57 patients (24 males, mean age 43.54±12.82 years) 30 healthy controls	Multiple drugs Prospective, 2 years	Hippocampus — Smaller bilateral hippocampal volume in male relapsing patients vs. healthy controls
Costafreda et al. [24]	37 patients (9 males, mean age 43.2±8.8 years) 37 healthy controls (9 males, mean age 42.8±6.7 years)	Fluoxetine, 20 mg/day Prospective, 8 weeks	Automated analysis — Larger GM volume in right rostral anterior cingulate cortex, left posterior cingulate cortex, left middle frontal gyrus, and right occipital cortex in remitted patients vs. nonremitted
Gunning et al. [35][a]	22 remitted patients (mean age 71.0±5.6 years) 19 nonremitted patients (mean age 70.0±6.3, years)	Escitalopram, 10 mg/day Prospective, 12 weeks	Anterior cingulate — Smaller dorsal and rostral anterior cingulate GM volumes in nonremitters vs. remitters
Li et al. [61]	25 nonremitted (5 males, mean age 46.5±10.4 years) 19 remitted (6 males, mean age 42.6±13.0 years)	Multiple drugs (SSRIs, SNRIs, or bupropion) Prospective, 6 weeks	Automated analysis — Smaller left DLPFC in nonremitters compared to remitters

(continued)

Table 15.1 (continued)

Author	Subjects	Treatment	Brain areas	Results
Lorenzetti et al. [63]	27 remitted patients (9 males, mean age 35,07±9,96 years) 29 currently ill patients (7 males, mean age 32,52±8,28 years) 31 healthy controls (10 males, mean age 34,68±9,86 years)	Multiple drugs Cross-sectional	Amygdala	Larger left amygdala volumes in remitted patients vs. healthy controls and currently ill patients
Sheline et al. [90][a]	217 patients (96 males, mean age 68.4±7.2 years)	Sertraline, up to 200 mg/day Prospective, 12 weeks	WM hyperintensities	Lower signal hyperintensities in remitters vs. nonremitters
Gunning-Dixon et al. [36][a]	22 remitted patients (9 males, 69.61±4.71 years) 20 nonremitted patients (8 males, 71.18±6.95 years) 25 healthy controls (9 males, 70.68±5.82 years)	Escitalopram, 10 mg/day Prospective, 12 weeks	Signal hyperintensities	Greater signal hyperintensities in nonremitters vs. healthy controls and remitters
Lai and Hsu [58]	15 patients (5 males, mean age 35.87±9.59, years) 15 healthy controls (4 males, mean age 34.30±9.87 years)	Duloxetine, 60 mg/day Longitudinal, 6 weeks	Automated analysis	F-up: Larger GM volumes over left inferior frontal cortex, right occipital fusiform gyrus, and right cerebellum VIIIa regions in remitted patients compared to baseline
Sneed et al. [94]	28 nonremitted patients (17 males, mean age 66.5±7.9 years) 10 remitted patients (5 males, mean age 64.7±6.5 years)	Sertraline, up to 200 mg/day Nortriptyline, 1 mg/kg/day Prospective, 12 weeks	WM hyperintensities	Greater hyperintensities in nonremitted patients vs. remitted patients

Sheline et al. [91][a]	168 patients (mean age 67.96 ± 7.49 years) 50 healthy controls (mean age 73.00 ± 5.31 years)	Sertraline, up to 200 mg/day Prospective, 12 weeks	Hippocampus, amygdala, parahippocampus, and caudate, anterior cingulate gyrus, frontal pole, superior frontal gyrus, orbital frontal gyrus, and middle frontal gyrus	Smaller hippocampal volume and frontal cortical thickness in nonremitters vs. remitters
Smith et al. [93]	13 patients (4 males, mean age 35.23 ± 9.04 years) 10 healthy controls (1 males, mean age 35.67 ± 12.3 years)	Sertraline, up to 200 mg/day Longitudinal, 12 weeks	Automated analysis	F-up: Enlargement in DLPFC in patients compared to baseline
Ribeiz et al. [83]	30 patients (7 males, mean age 70.73 ± 6.59 years) 22 patients (5 males, mean age 70.41 ± 7.58)	Not specified antidepressant treatment Prospective, 24 weeks	Automated analysis	Larger left lateral OFC in remitted patients vs. nonremitted
Kong et al. [54]	28 drug-naive patients (11 males, mean age 34.42 ± 8.24 years) 28 healthy controls (14 males, mean age 32.07 ± 9.27 years) 24 treated patients acquired at f-up (10 males, mean age 36.12 ± 5.73 years)	Fluoxetine, 10 – 40 mg/day Longitudinal, 8 weeks	Automated analysis	Larger left middle frontal gyrus and right OFC in treated patients at f-up vs. healthy controls No differences between drug-naive and treated patients

(continued)

Table 15.1 (continued)

Author	Subjects	Treatment	Brain areas	Results
Yuen et al. [105]	16 patients with apathy (7 males, mean age 71.6±5 years) 29 patients without apathy (10 males, 69±5.8 years) 49 healthy controls (16 males, mean age 70.6±6.4 years)	Escitalopram 10 mg Prospective, 12 weeks	Cingulate cortex	Larger left posterior subgenual cingulate volume correlated with apathy amelioration
Taylor et al. [96]	11 patients (5 males, mean age 64.6±4.4 years)	Citalopram fluoxetine, sertraline, venlafaxine Prospective 3 and 6 months	WM hyperintensities	Greater WM hyperintensities at cingulum bundle associated with worse outcome
Jung et al. [48]	26 nonresponders (7 males, mean age 40.8±12.7 years) 24 responders (7 males, mean age 43.0±10.1 years) 29 healthy controls (8 males, mean age 43.6±13.4 years)	Bupropion, duloxetine, escitalopram, venlafaxine, paroxetine Prospective, 8 weeks	Automated analysis	Smaller right superior frontal gyrus in nonremitters Larger lingual gyrus in remitters
Korgaonkar et al. [55]	40 nonresponders (males 19, mean age 37.1±14.8 years) 34 responders (18 males, mean age 28.2±7.4 years)	Escitalopram, sertraline, venlafaxine Prospective, 8 weeks	Automated analysis	Smaller left middle frontal gyrus and larger right angular gyrus in nonremitters
Klauser et al. [52]	29 patients currently ill (7 males, mean age 33.09±8.25 years) 27 remitted patients (9 males, mean age 35.02±9.72 years)	Multiple treatments (SSRIs, SNRIs, TCAs, NsSSAs, MAOIs, NRIs) Cross-sectional	Automated analysis	No treatment effect

| Fu et al. [30] | 32 patients (19 males, mean age 42.2±11.2 years) 25 healthy controls (12 males, mean age 38.8±9.9 years) | Duloxetine 60–120 mg Longitudinal, 8 weeks | MR scan 0, 1, 8, 12 weeks Amygdala, anterior cingulate, hippocampus | Larger hippocampal volumes among remitters |
| Phillips et al. [80] | 14 remitted patients (3 males, mean age 44.7±10.5 years) 12 remitted (5 males, mean age 47.5±10.6 years) | Multiple treatments Longitudinal, 6 months from remission to 12 months of nonremission | Hippocampus, rostral middle frontal gyrus, orbitofrontal cortex, rostral and caudal anterior cingulate cortices, and inferior temporal gyrus | Larger hippocampal volume and cortical thickness in the rostral middle frontal gyrus, orbitofrontal cortex, and inferior temporal gyrus in remitters vs. nonremitters |

Legend: DLPFC dorsolateral prefrontal cortex, *f-up* follow-up, *GM* gray matter, *HDRS* hamilton depression rating Scale, *WM* white matter, *OFC* orbitofrontal cortex
aOverlapping samples

5.3   Magnetic Resonance Alterations in Depressive Illness (Table 15.1)

Even though the neurobiology of depression has not yet completely understood, brain structural alterations have been reported in frontotemporal, hippocampal, and striatal regions [1]. Clinical depression includes different domains that involve cognitive, emotional, and neurovegetative symptoms. Neurobiological hypotheses on the etiopathology of this heterogeneous syndrome involve stress response mechanisms, immunomodulatory impairment, and neurochemical alterations. Thus, brain area alteration studies have been focused on those circuits, which are implicated in stress-related response or on those neurotransmitters such as serotonin and norepinephrine, which have been selected as target biochemicals for antidepressant treatment. Evidence in this field is still inconclusive and brain imaging offers a valid and widely available instrument to investigate the neurobiological implications of the disease and the mechanism of action of effective therapies [9]. Also, imaging results can differentiate groups of patients who respond to antidepressant therapies from those who do not. Indeed, rates of treatment response to antidepressants reach about 30 %, even after multiple trials. Enrollment of patients with treatment resistance due to not yet recognized cause might limit the power of drug trials to demonstrate efficacy of new compounds; furthermore, time spent on inefficacious treatments causes a delay in the consideration of more efficacious approaches for refractory patients. For these reasons, ability to predict treatment response is a challenge for the progression of research on novel treatments for depression. In this field, imaging features can offer an objective and replicable predictor of treatment efficacy or response.

Imaging studies on depressive disorder have often focused on limbic system structures, namely, hippocampus and amygdala, since they are involved in functions such as declarative memory and mood regulation, which are impaired in depression. Converging evidence from animal postmortem and clinical examinations reports reduction of volumes in hippocampus in depressive disorder. MR data confirm robustly this observation. Hippocampi have been reported to be reduced in volume in patients with chronic depression [22, 44], nonremitting, first episode, or unmedicated patients [5], with only few contrary results of no volume change in comparison with healthy controls [102]. Lower volumes were reported to progress over time [28, 29]; duration of illness, rather than age, has been hypothesized to determine hippocampal volume reduction. As these results were observed in a heterogeneous population, several hypotheses have been raised to explain lower hippocampal volumes in depression. The connection between stress, hypercortisolemia, and hippocampal function has often been sustained, not only by imaging studies [66]. However, factors such as illness duration, long-term pharmacological treatment, life events (e.g., sexual or childhood abuse [101]), comorbidity with anxiety disorders, somatoform disorders, or alcohol (substance) abuse [95] might have confounded results in this field. The object has been summarized in few meta-analyses since the early 2000s. Campbell and colleagues reported reduced hippocampal volume in patients with depressive disorder [13]. Inconsistencies across studies have been attributed to methodological issues such as slice thickness of images, due to differences in the machinery adopted, or tracing methods, or definition of anatomical boundaries of hippocampus (particularly the limit between hippocampus and amygdala). Indeed, the shape rather than the overall volume of hippocampus might be altered, as effect of fibers' disruption [12]. Duration of illness has been accounted for one of the major contributors to hippocampal atrophy, which have been observed in schizophrenia as well [12]. Nevertheless, reduction of volume has been confirmed for patients at first depression episode [21]. These data have been further confirmed by Arnone and colleagues [1].

Along with hippocampus, a reduction of volume has been frequently observed for amygdala, also [89]. Reduction of volume has been reported for psychotic, recent-onset, and chronic depression [39]. Recent meta-analyses have been reviewed the opinion of a reduction of volume in the amygdala among patients with depression; they concluded there's not a volume reduction in amygdala [13] and argued that inconsistency across studies can be related to either technical variables, such as different anatomical boundaries adopted for selecting the area, or slice thickness, or biological variables, such as administration of pharmacological treatment or age or illness duration [1]. Even though structural imaging did not demonstrate a consistent structural alteration in the amygdala among patients with depression, the structure is still considered to have an important implication in the illness. This assumption has been robustly confirmed by functional, rather than structural, imaging studies which reported an altered activation of amygdala during affective tasks and a "retuning" of its activity after successful pharmacological treatment [9].

Cortical alterations have been observed in temporal and frontal lobes in depressive disorder. Prefrontal and orbitofrontal cortex reduction of volume, along with anterior cingulate cortex, have been reported in geriatric as well as recent-onset depression. Specifically, lower gray matter (GM) gyrification index has been observed in prefrontal and anterior cingulate cortex. These alterations have been reported by longitudinal studies to undergo a progressive process, faster than normal aging degeneration [29]. Nevertheless, findings on prefrontal areas are sometimes inconclusive [52], particularly for anterior cingulate [11], though its functional implication in depression has been robustly reported [81]. Heterogeneity of results should take into account differences in illness severity or time course, gender, anatomical variability, or tracing protocols.

Reduction of volume in temporal lobe for severe patients or reduced cortical thickness in recent onset [99] has been reported for some studies even though some results report unaltered volumes [76]. Probably, lateralization (left volume reduction more than right) and duration of illness affect the results [102]. Furthermore, white matter (WM) alterations (hyperintensities) have been observed, mostly in geriatric population [86, 87] but also in first episode, specifically in the corpus callosum. Finally, basal ganglia alterations, such as volume reduction or signal hyperintensities, have been reported, in the caudate, the putamen, globus pallidus, and in the neighboring thalamus.

5.3.1 Features of Treatment Response

Along with structural alterations related to depressive disorder, imaging studies have also investigated structural features of treatment response in terms of effect of single compounds or predictors of treatment response. Only few studies have observed the effect of antidepressant administration over time in a longitudinal design. Increased hippocampal volume and cortical thickness in the rostral middle frontal gyrus, orbitofrontal cortex, and inferior temporal gyrus in remitters and decreased volume or thickness in these regions in nonremitters were observed after 6–12 months of observation after multiple antidepressant treatments [80]. First episode patients with major depression (MD), medication naive, under short-term administration of fluoxetine, showed larger volumes in prefrontal areas – middle frontal gyrus and orbitofrontal cortex – compared to healthy controls, along with treatment response [54]. Sertraline administration determined enlargement of volume of dorsolateral prefrontal cortex (DLPFC) among responsive MD patients, compared to healthy controls [93]. Also, among drug-naive patients with MD, duloxetine treatment determined amelioration of inferofrontal areas shrinkage, observed at baseline, in comparison to healthy controls; enlargement came along with clinical improvement but did not reach the same volume of healthy controls [58]. In a different sample, 12 weeks administration of duloxetine was not associated with structural changes but with increased functional connectivity in prefrontal areas [30]. These data underlie the implication of prefrontal area structural remodeling during response to treatment [59], probably associated with a cortical modulatory effect on emotional neuronal circuits. Indeed, larger prefrontal area volumes and cortical thickness, in middle frontal gyrus, DLPFC, or anterior cingulate, have been reported as predictors of better clinical outcome, in prospective studies [19, 24, 35, 48, 55, 60, 63]: these studies assessed patients only ones and test structural imaging predictors of treatment response after few weeks of treatment. In a sample of geriatric patients, larger anterior cingulate orbitofrontal cortex volume predicted lower levels of apathy after 12 weeks of escitalopram administration [105] or clinical remission [83]. Among geriatric populations, a predictive negative effect of white matter hyperintensities on treatment outcome was observed [36, 78, 90, 94], particularly for cingulate fibers [96].

Several predictive reports have focused on hippocampus, in terms of identification of markers of treatment response, because it is considered as a core area for the pathophysiology of depressive disorder and its volumetric reduction has been correlated to illness severity and poor outcome [73, 100]. Larger hippocampal volume predicted treatment response to antidepressants [30, 64, 91], whereas nonremitting patients had lower volumes at baseline and did not undergo an increase of volume at follow-up, whereas those who respond had larger volume compared to baseline [29]. Hippocampus volumetric response to antidepressant treatment, along with clinical improvement, might be more evident in female patients, suggesting a possible gender effect.

5.4 Summary

The growing recognition of personalized medicine in psychiatry not only by clinicians and researchers but also politicians, patients, and the pharmaceutical industry reflects the need for an improvement of diagnostic processes and therapeutic algorithms. Biomarkers are supposed to improve and expand the diagnostic options and enable patient-tailored treatments. Despite great efforts, imaging biomarkers are still not sensitive nor specific enough to allow the application in clinical practice. However, they offer valid landmarks on the neurobiological substrates of psychiatric diseases. The main imaging findings suggest an altered brain network that encompasses the anterior cingulate, the prefrontal cortex, and the hippocampus in major depression. Few studies have addressed the effects of pharmacological treatment on brain structures. Most of them offer hints of features of treatment response rather than explaining differential neural effects of single compounds. Antidepressants, mainly the SSRIs, might exert neuroprotective effects, which determine a reduction of hippocampal and prefrontal cortex shrinkage, probably through an activation of neuromodulatory factors like BDNF. Altered levels of BDNF belong also to the most replicated findings in the field of blood-based biomarkers. Lower BDNF plasma levels are observed in depressed patients and normalize after successful treatment. Even though the development of blood-based biomarkers in psychiatric disorders is still in its infancy, there are some very promising findings observed within inflammatory pathways and the HPA axis. In both systems, there is accumulating evidence that drugs specifically targeting these systems may be beneficial for the treatment of depression, but only in these patients who have marked alterations detected by the respective biomarkers.

Acknowledgments PB was partially supported by grants from the Italian Ministry of Health (RF-2011-02352308), the BIAL Foundation (Fellowship#262/12), and the IRCCS "E. Medea" (Ricerca Corrente).

AM inventor: Means and methods for diagnosing predisposition for treatment emergent suicidal ideation (TESI). *European patent number: 2166112. International application number: PCT/EP2009/061575.*

References

1. Arnone D, McIntosh AM, Ebmeier KP, Munafo MR, Anderson IM (2012) Magnetic resonance imaging studies in unipolar depression: systematic review and meta-regression analyses. Eur Neuropsychopharmacol 22(1):1–16. doi:10.1016/j.euroneuro.2011.05.003
2. Aschbacher K, Mills PJ, von Kanel R, Hong S, Mausbach BT, Roepke SK, Dimsdale JE, Patterson TL, Ziegler MG, Ancoli-Israel S, Grant I (2008) Effects of depressive and anxious symptoms on norepinephrine and platelet P-selectin responses to acute psychological stress among elderly caregivers. Brain Behav Immun 22(4):493–502. doi:10.1016/j.bbi.2007.10.002
3. Aubry JM N, Osiek C, Perret G, Rossier MF, Bertschy G, Bondolfi G (2007) The DEX/CRH neuroendocrine test and the prediction of depressive relapse in remitted depressed outpatients. JPsychiatrRes41(3–4):290–294.doi:10.1016/j.jpsychires.2006.07.007,S0022-3956(06)00143-9 [pii]

4. Barron E, Lara J, White M, Mathers JC (2015) Blood-borne biomarkers of mortality risk: systematic review of cohort studies. PLoS One 10(6):e0127550. doi:10.1371/journal. pone.0127550
5. Bearden CE, Thompson PM, Avedissian C, Klunder AD, Nicoletti M, Dierschke N, Brambilla P, Soares JC (2009) Altered hippocampal morphology in unmedicated patients with major depressive illness. ASN Neuro 1(4). doi:AN20090026 [pii] 10.1042/AN20090026
6. Belanoff JK, Rothschild AJ, Cassidy F, DeBattista C, Baulieu EE, Schold C, Schatzberg AF (2002) An open label trial of C-1073 (mifepristone) for psychotic major depression. Biol Psychiatry 52(5):386–392
7. Bellani M, Dusi N, Brambilla P (2010) Longitudinal imaging studies in schizophrenia: the relationship between brain morphology and outcome measures. Epidemiol Psichiatr Soc 19(3):207–210
8. Bellani M, Dusi N, Brambilla P (2013) Can brain imaging address psychosocial functioning and outcome in schizophrenia? In: Thornicroft G, Ruggeri M, Goldberg D (eds) Improving mental health care: the global challenge. Wiley-Blackwell, pp 281–290
9. Bellani M, Dusi N, Yeh PH, Soares JC, Brambilla P (2011) The effects of antidepressants on human brain as detected by imaging studies. Focus on major depression. Prog Neuropsychopharmacol Biol Psychiatry 35(7):1544–1552. doi:10.1016/j.pnpbp.2010.11.040
10. Binder EB (2009) The role of FKBP5, a co-chaperone of the glucocorticoid receptor in the pathogenesis and therapy of affective and anxiety disorders. Psychoneuroendocrinology 34(Suppl 1):186–195. doi:10.1016/j.psyneuen.2009.05.021, S0306-4530(09)00185-1 [pii]
11. Brambilla P, Nicoletti MA, Harenski K, Sassi RB, Mallinger AG, Frank E, Kupfer DJ, Keshavan MS, Soares JC (2002) Anatomical MRI study of subgenual prefrontal cortex in bipolar and unipolar subjects. Neuropsychopharmacology 27(5):792–799. doi:10.1016/S0893-133X(02)00352-4
12. Brambilla P, Perlini C, Rajagopalan P, Saharan P, Rambaldelli G, Bellani M, Dusi N, Cerini R, Pozzi Mucelli R, Tansella M, Thompson PM (2013) Schizophrenia severity, social functioning and hippocampal neuroanatomy: three-dimensional mapping study. Br J Psychiatry 202(1):50–55. doi:10.1192/bjp.bp.111.105700
13. Campbell S, Marriott M, Nahmias C, MacQueen GM (2004) Lower hippocampal volume in patients suffering from depression: a meta-analysis. Am J Psychiatry 161(4):598–607
14. Carpenter LL, Ross NS, Tyrka AR, Anderson GM, Kelly M, Price LH (2009) Dex/CRH test cortisol response in outpatients with major depression and matched healthy controls. Psychoneuroendocrinology 34(8):1208–1213. doi:10.1016/j.psyneuen.2009.03.009, S0306-4530(09)00092-4 [pii]
15. Carroll BJ, Curtis GC, Mendels J (1976) Neuroendocrine regulation in depression. II. Discrimination of depressed from nondepressed patients. Arch Gen Psychiatry 33(9):1051–1058
16. Cattaneo A, Bocchio-Chiavetto L, Zanardini R, Milanesi E, Placentino A, Gennarelli M (2010) Reduced peripheral brain-derived neurotrophic factor mRNA levels are normalized by antidepressant treatment. Int J Neuropsychopharmacol 13(1):103–108. doi:10.1017/S1461145709990812, S1461145709990812 [pii]
17. Cattaneo A, Gennarelli M, Uher R, Breen G, Farmer A, Aitchison KJ, Craig IW, Anacker C, Zunsztain PA, McGuffin P, Pariante CM (2013) Candidate genes expression profile associated with antidepressants response in the GENDEP study: differentiating between baseline 'predictors' and longitudinal 'targets'. Neuropsychopharmacology 38(3):377–385. doi:10.1038/npp.2012.191, npp2012191 [pii]
18. Cattaneo A, Sesta A, Calabrese F, Nielsen G, Riva MA, Gennarelli M (2013) The expression of VGF is reduced in leukocytes of depressed patients and it is restored by effective antidepressant treatment. Neuropsychopharmacology 35(7):1423–1428. doi:10.1038/npp.2010.11, npp201011 [pii]
19. Chen CH, Ridler K, Suckling J, Williams S, Fu CH, Merlo-Pich E, Bullmore E (2007) Brain imaging correlates of depressive symptom severity and predictors of symptom improvement after antidepressant treatment. Biological psychiatry 62(5):407–414. doi:10.1016/j.biopsych.2006.09.018

20. Clark-Raymond A, Meresh E, Hoppensteadt D, Fareed J, Sinacore J, Halaris A (2014) Vascular Endothelial Growth Factor: a potential diagnostic biomarker for major depression. J Psychiatr Res 59:22–27. doi:10.1016/j.jpsychires.2014.08.005
21. Cole J, Costafreda SG, McGuffin P, Fu CH (2011) Hippocampal atrophy in first episode depression: a meta-analysis of magnetic resonance imaging studies. J Affect Disord 134(1–3):483–487. doi:10.1016/j.jad.2011.05.057
22. Colla M, Kronenberg G, Deuschle M, Meichel K, Hagen T, Bohrer M, Heuser I (2007) Hippocampal volume reduction and HPA-system activity in major depression. J Psychiatr Res 41(7):553–560. doi:10.1016/j.jpsychires.2006.06.011
23. Coryell W, Schlesser M (2001) The dexamethasone suppression test and suicide prediction. Am J Psychiatry 158(5):748–753.
24. Costafreda SG, Chu C, Ashburner J, Fu CH (2009) Prognostic and diagnostic potential of the structural neuroanatomy of depression. PloS one 4(7):e6353. doi:10.1371/journal.pone.0006353
25. Dusi N, Perlini C, Bellani M, Brambilla P (2012) Searching for psychosocial endophenotypes in schizophrenia: the innovative role of brain imaging. Riv Psichiatr 47(2):76–88. doi:10.1708/1069.11712
26. Fernandes BS, Berk M, Turck CW, Steiner J, Goncalves CA (2014) Decreased peripheral brain-derived neurotrophic factor levels are a biomarker of disease activity in major psychiatric disorders: a comparative meta-analysis. Mol Psychiatry 19(7):750–751. doi:10.1038/mp.2013.172
27. Flores BH, Kenna H, Keller J, Solvason HB, Schatzberg AF (2006) Clinical and biological effects of mifepristone treatment for psychotic depression. Neuropsychopharmacology 31(3):628–636. doi:10.1038/sj.npp.1300884
28. Frodl T, Meisenzahl EM, Zetzsche T, Hohne T, Banac S, Schorr C, Jager M, Leinsinger G, Bottlender R, Reiser M, Moller HJ (2004) Hippocampal and amygdala changes in patients with major depressive disorder and healthy controls during a 1-year follow-up. The Journal of clinical psychiatry 65(4):492–499
29. Frodl TS, Koutsouleris N, Bottlender R, Born C, Jager M, Scupin I, Reiser M, Moller HJ, Meisenzahl EM (2008) Depression-related variation in brain morphology over 3 years: effects of stress? Arch Gen Psychiatry 65(10):1156–1165. doi:10.1001/archpsyc.65.10.1156
30. Fu C, Costafreda S, Sankar A, Adams T, Rasenick M, Liu P, Donati R, Maglanoc L, Horton P, Marangell L (2015) Multimodal functional and structural neuroimaging investigation of major depressive disorder following treatment with duloxetine. BMC Psychiatry 15(1):82
31. Gaali S, Kirschner A, Cuboni S, Hartmann J, Kozany C, Balsevich G, Namendorf C, Fernandez-Vizarra P, Sippel C, Zannas AS, Draenert R, Binder EB, Almeida OF, Ruhter G, Uhr M, Schmidt MV, Touma C, Bracher A, Hausch F (2015) Selective inhibitors of the FK506-binding protein 51 by induced fit. Nat Chem Biol 11(1):33–37. doi:10.1038/nchembio.1699
32. Galfalvy H, Currier D, Oquendo MA, Sullivan G, Huang YY, John Mann J (2009) Lower CSF MHPG predicts short-term risk for suicide attempt. Int J Neuropsychopharmacol 12(10):1327–1335. doi:10.1017/S1461145709990228
33. Gallagher P, Malik N, Newham J, Young AH, Ferrier IN, Mackin P (2015) WITHDRAWN: Antiglucocorticoid treatments for mood disorders. Cochrane Database Syst Rev 6:CD005168. doi:10.1002/14651858.CD005168.pub3
34. Gold PW (2015) The organization of the stress system and its dysregulation in depressive illness. Mol Psychiatry 20(1):32–47. doi:10.1038/mp.2014.163
35. Gunning FM, Cheng J, Murphy CF, Kanellopoulos D, Acuna J, Hoptman MJ, Klimstra S, Morimoto S, Weinberg J, Alexopoulos GS (2009) Anterior cingulate cortical volumes and treatment remission of geriatric depression. International Journal of Geriatric Psychiatry 24(8):829–836. doi:10.1002/gps.2290
36. Gunning-Dixon FM, Walton M, Cheng J, Acuna J, Klimstra S, Zimmerman ME, Brickman AM, Hoptman MJ, Young RC, Alexopoulos GS (2010) MRI signal hyperintensities and treatment remission of geriatric depression. Journal of Affective Disorders 126(3):395–401. doi:http://dx.doi.org/10.1016/j.jad.2010.04.004

37. Halmai Z, Dome P, Dobos J, Gonda X, Szekely A, Sasvari-Szekely M, Faludi G, Lazary J (2013) Peripheral vascular endothelial growth factor level is associated with antidepressant treatment response: results of a preliminary study. J Affect Disord 144(3):269–273. doi:10.1016/j.jad.2012.09.006
38. Harley J, Luty S, Carter J, Mulder R, Joyce P (2010) Elevated C-reactive protein in depression: a predictor of good long-term outcome with antidepressants and poor outcome with psychotherapy. J Psychopharmacol 24(4):625–626. doi:10.1177/0269881109102770
39. Hastings RS, Parsey RV, Oquendo MA, Arango V, Mann JJ (2004) Volumetric analysis of the prefrontal cortex, amygdala, and hippocampus in major depression. Neuropsychopharmacology 29(5):952–959. doi:10.1038/sj.npp.1300371
40. Hennings JM, Uhr M, Klengel T, Weber P, Putz B, Touma C, Czamara D, Ising M, Holsboer F, Lucae S (2015) RNA expression profiling in depressed patients suggests retinoid-related orphan receptor alpha as a biomarker for antidepressant response. Transcult Psychiatry 5:e538. doi:10.1038/tp.2015.9
41. Heuser I, Yassouridis A, Holsboer F (1994) The combined dexamethasone/CRH test: a refined laboratory test for psychiatric disorders. J Psychiatr Res 28(4):341–356
42. Himmerich H, Fulda S, Sheldrick AJ, Plumakers B, Rink L (2010) IFN-gamma reduction by tricyclic antidepressants. Int J Psychiatry Med 40(4):413–424
43. Holsboer F (2000) The corticosteroid receptor hypothesis of depression. Neuropsychopharmacology 23(5):477–501
44. Hsieh MH, McQuoid DR, Levy RM, Payne ME, MacFall JR, Steffens DC (2002) Hippocampal volume and antidepressant response in geriatric depression. International Journal of Geriatric Psychiatry 17(6):519–525. doi:10.1002/gps.611
45. Ising M, Horstmann S, Kloiber S, Lucae S, Binder EB, Kern N, Kunzel HE, Pfennig A, Uhr M, Holsboer F (2007) Combined dexamethasone/corticotropin releasing hormone test predicts treatment response in major depression – a potential biomarker? Biol Psychiatry 62(1):47–54. doi:10.1016/j.biopsych.2006.07.039 , S0006-3223(06)01002-X [pii]
46. Iyengar RL, Gandhi S, Aneja A, Thorpe K, Razzouk L, Greenberg J, Mosovich S, Farkouh ME (2013) NSAIDs are associated with lower depression scores in patients with osteoarthritis. Am J Med 126(11):1017 e1011–1018. doi:10.1016/j.amjmed.2013.02.037
47. Jetten AM (2004) Recent advances in the mechanisms of action and physiological functions of the retinoid-related orphan receptors (RORs). Curr Drug Targets Inflamm Allergy 3(4):395–412
48. Jung J, Kang J, Won E, Nam K, Lee M-S, Tae WS, Ham B-J (2014) Impact of lingual gyrus volume on antidepressant response and neurocognitive functions in Major Depressive Disorder: A voxel-based morphometry study. Journal of Affective Disorders 169:179–187. doi:http://dx.doi.org/10.1016/j.jad.2014.08.018
49. Kaestner F, Hettich M, Peters M, Sibrowski W, Hetzel G, Ponath G, Arolt V, Cassens U, Rothermundt M (2005) Different activation patterns of proinflammatory cytokines in melancholic and non-melancholic major depression are associated with HPA axis activity. J Affect Disord 87(2–3):305–311. doi:10.1016/j.jad.2005.03.012 , S0165-0327(05)00087-X [pii]
50. Kapczinski F, Dal-Pizzol F, Teixeira AL, Magalhaes PV, Kauer-Sant'Anna M, Klamt F, Pasquali MA, Quevedo J, Gama CS, Post R (2010) A systemic toxicity index developed to assess peripheral changes in mood episodes. Mol Psychiatry 15(8):784–786. doi:10.1038/mp.2009.112
51. Katz ER, Stowe ZN, Newport DJ, Kelley ME, Pace TW, Cubells JF, Binder EB (2012) Regulation of mRNA expression encoding chaperone and co-chaperone proteins of the glucocorticoid receptor in peripheral blood: association with depressive symptoms during pregnancy. Psychol Med 42(5):943–956. doi:10.1017/S0033291711002121, S0033291711002121 [pii]
52. Klauser P, Fornito A, Lorenzetti V, Davey CG, Dwyer DB, Allen NB, Yücel M (2015) Cortico-limbic network abnormalities in individuals with current and past major depressive disorder. J Affect Disord 173(0):45–52. doi:http://dx.doi.org/10.1016/j.jad.2014.10.041
53. Kohler O, Benros ME, Nordentoft M, Farkouh ME, Iyengar RL, Mors O, Krogh J (2014) Effect of anti-inflammatory treatment on depression, depressive symptoms, and adverse

effects: a systematic review and meta-analysis of randomized clinical trials. JAMA Psychiatry 71(12):1381–1391. doi:10.1001/jamapsychiatry.2014.1611

54. Kong L, Wu F, Tang Y, Ren L, Kong D, Liu Y, Xu K, Wang F (2014) Frontal-subcortical volumetric deficits in single episode, medication-naive depressed patients and the effects of 8 weeks fluoxetine treatment: a VBM-DARTEL study. PLoS One 9(1):e79055. doi:10.1371/journal.pone.0079055

55. Korgaonkar MS, Rekshan W, Gordon E, Rush AJ, Williams LM, Blasey C, Grieve SM (2015) Magnetic resonance imaging measures of brain structure to predict antidepressant treatment outcome in major depressive disorder. EBioMedicine 2(1):37–45. doi:10.1016/j.ebiom.2014.12.002

56. Kronmuller KT, Pantel J, Gotz B, Kohler S, Victor D, Mundt C, Magnotta VA, Giesel F, Essig M, Schroder J (2008) Life events and hippocampal volume in first-episode major depression. J Affect Disord. 110:241–7

57. Kunugi H, Ida I, Owashi T, Kimura M, Inoue Y, Nakagawa S, Yabana T, Urushibara T, Kanai R, Aihara M, Yuuki N, Otsubo T, Oshima A, Kudo K, Inoue T, Kitaichi Y, Shirakawa O, Isogawa K, Nagayama H, Kamijima K, Nanko S, Kanba S, Higuchi T, Mikuni M (2006) Assessment of the Dexamethasone/CRH test as a state-dependent marker for hypothalamic-pituitary-adrenal (HPA) axis abnormalities in major depressive episode: a multicenter study. Neuropsychopharmacology 31(1):212–220

58. Lai C, Hsu, YY (2011) A subtle grey-matter increase in first-episode, drug-naive major depressive disorder with panic disorder after 6 weeks' duloxetine therapy. Int J Neuropsychopharmacol. 14:225–35

59. Lavretsky H, Roybal DJ, Ballmaier M, Toga AW, Kumar A (2005) Antidepressant exposure may protect against decrement in frontal gray matter volumes in geriatric depression. The Journal of Clinical Psychiatry 66(8):964–967

60. Liew CC, Ma J, Tang HC, Zheng R, Dempsey AA (2006) The peripheral blood transcriptome dynamically reflects system wide biology: a potential diagnostic tool. J Lab Clin Med 147:126–132

61. Li C-T, Lin C-P, Chou K-H, Chen IY, Hsieh J-C, Wu C-L, Lin W-C, Su T-P (2010) Structural and cognitive deficits in remitting and non-remitting recurrent depression: A voxel-based morphometric study. NeuroImage 50(1):347–356. doi:http://dx.doi.org/10.1016/j.neuroimage.2009.11.021

62. Liu Y, Ho RC, Mak A (2012) Interleukin (IL)-6, tumour necrosis factor alpha (TNF-alpha) and soluble interleukin-2 receptors (sIL-2R) are elevated in patients with major depressive disorder: a meta-analysis and meta-regression. J Affect Disord 139(3):230–239. doi:10.1016/j.jad.2011.08.003

63. Lorenzetti V, Allen NB, Whittle S, Yücel M (2010) Amygdala volumes in a sample of current depressed and remitted depressed patients and healthy controls. Journal of Affective Disorders 120(1–3):112–119. doi:http://dx.doi.org/10.1016/j.jad.2009.04.021

64. MacQueen GM, Yucel K, Taylor VH, Macdonald K, Joffe R (2008) Posterior Hippocampal Volumes Are Associated with Remission Rates in Patients with Major Depressive Disorder. Biological Psychiatry 64(10):880–883. doi:http://dx.doi.org/10.1016/j.biopsych.2008.06.027

65. Matsubara T, Funato H, Kobayashi A, Nobumoto M, Watanabe Y (2006) Reduced glucocorticoid receptor alpha expression in mood disorder patients and first-degree relatives. Biol Psychiatry 59(8):689–695. doi:10.1016/j.biopsych.2005.09.026, S0006-3223(05)01431-9 [pii]

66. McEwen BS (2000) Effects of adverse experiences for brain structure and function. Biol Psychiatry 48(8):721–731

67. Menke A, Arloth J, Gerber M, Rex-Haffner M, Uhr M, Holsboer F, Binder EB, Holsboer-Trachsler E, Beck J (2014) Dexamethasone stimulated gene expression in peripheral blood indicates glucocorticoid-receptor hypersensitivity in job-related exhaustion. Psychoneuroendocrinology 44:35–46. doi:10.1016/j.psyneuen.2014.02.013, S0306-4530(14)00064-X [pii]

68. Menke A, Arloth J, Putz B, Weber P, Klengel T, Mehta D, Gonik M, Rex-Haffner M, Rubel J, Uhr M, Lucae S, Deussing JM, Muller-Myhsok B, Holsboer F, Binder EB (2012) Dexamethasone stimulated gene expression in peripheral blood is a sensitive marker for glu-

cocorticoid receptor resistance in depressed patients. Neuropsychopharmacology 37(6):1455–1464. doi:10.1038/npp.2011.331, npp2011331 [pii]

69. Menke A, Klengel T, Rubel J, Bruckl T, Pfister H, Lucae S, Uhr M, Holsboer F, Binder EB (2013) Genetic variation in FKBP5 associated with the extent of stress hormone dysregulation in major depression. Genes Brain Behav 12(3):289–296. doi:10.1111/gbb.12026

70. Murphy GM Jr, Sarginson JE, Ryan HS, O'Hara R, Schatzberg AF, Lazzeroni LC (2013) BDNF and CREB1 genetic variants interact to affect antidepressant treatment outcomes in geriatric depression. Pharmacogenet Genomics 23(6):301–313. doi:10.1097/FPC.0b013e328360b175, 01213011–201306000–00002 [pii]

71. Na KS, Lee KJ, Lee JS, Cho YS, Jung HY (2014) Efficacy of adjunctive celecoxib treatment for patients with major depressive disorder: a meta-analysis. Prog Neuropsychopharmacol Biol Psychiatry 48:79–85. doi:10.1016/j.pnpbp.2013.09.006

72. Nelson JC, Davis JM (1997) DST studies in psychotic depression: a meta-analysis. Am J Psychiatry 154(11):1497–1503. doi:10.1038/nrcardio.2012.91

73. Neumeister A, Wood S, Bonne O, Nugent AC, Luckenbaugh DA, Young T, Bain EE, Charney DS, Drevets WC (2005) Reduced hippocampal volume in unmedicated, remitted patients with major depression versus control subjects. Biol Psychiatry 57(8):935–937. doi:10.1016/j.biopsych.2005.01.016

74. Nierenberg AA, Feinstein AR (1988) How to evaluate a diagnostic marker test. Lessons from the rise and fall of dexamethasone suppression test. JAMA 259(11):1699–1702

75. Pandey GN, Dwivedi Y, Rizavi HS, Ren X, Zhang H, Pavuluri MN (2010) Brain-derived neurotrophic factor gene and protein expression in pediatric and adult depressed subjects. Prog Neuropsychopharmacol Biol Psychiatry 34(4):645–651. doi:10.1016/j.pnpbp.2010.03.003, S0278–5846(10)00079–5 [pii]

76. Pantel J, Schröder J, Essig M, Popp D, Dech H, Knopp MV, Schad LR, Eysenbach K, Backenstraß M, Friedlinger M (1997) Quantitative magnetic resonance imaging in geriatric depression and primary degenerative dementia. J Affect Disord 42(1):69–83. doi:http://dx.doi.org/10.1016/S0165–0327(96)00105-X

77. Papakostas GI, Iosifescu DV, Renshaw PF, Lyoo IK, Lee HK, Alpert JE, Nierenberg AA, Fava M (2005) Brain MRI white matter hyperintensities and one-carbon cycle metabolism in non-geriatric outpatients with major depressive disorder (Part II). Psychiatry Research: Neuroimaging 140(3):301–307. doi:http://dx.doi.org/10.1016/j.pscychresns.2005.09.001

78. Paslakis G, Krumm B, Gilles M, Schweiger U, Heuser I, Richter I, Deuschle M (2011) Discrimination between patients with melancholic depression and healthy controls: comparison between 24-h cortisol profiles, the DST and the Dex/CRH test. Psychoneuroendocrinology 36(5):691–698. doi:10.1016/j.psyneuen.2010.10.002

79. Pfennig A, Kunzel HE, Kern N, Ising M, Majer M, Fuchs B, Ernst G, Holsboer F, Binder EB (2005) Hypothalamus-pituitary-adrenal system regulation and suicidal behavior in depression. Biol Psychiatry 57(4):336–342

80. Phillips JL, Batten LA, Tremblay P, Aldosary F, Blier P (2015) A prospective, longitudinal study of the effect of remission on cortical thickness and Hippocampal volume in patients with treatment-resistant depression. Int J Neuropsychopharmacol 18(8)

81. Pizzagalli DA, Oakes TR, Fox AS, Chung MK, Larson CL, Abercrombie HC, Schaefer SM, Benca RM, Davidson RJ (2004) Functional but not structural subgenual prefrontal cortex abnormalities in melancholia. Molecular psychiatry 9(4):325, 393–405. doi:10.1038/sj.mp.4001469

82. Raison CL, Rutherford RE, Woolwine BJ, Shuo C, Schettler P, Drake DF, Haroon E, Miller AH (2013) A randomized controlled trial of the tumor necrosis factor antagonist infliximab for treatment-resistant depression: the role of baseline inflammatory biomarkers. JAMA Psychiatry 70(1):31–41. doi:10.1001/2013.jamapsychiatry.4

83. Ribeiz SR, Duran F, Oliveira MC, Bezerra D, Castro CC, Steffens DC, Busatto Filho G, Bottino CM (2013) Structural brain changes as biomarkers and outcome predictors in patients with late-life depression: a cross-sectional and prospective study. PLoS One 8(11):e80049. doi:10.1371/journal.pone.0080049

84. Rupprecht R, Rupprecht M, Rupprecht C, Sofic E, Barocka A, Beck G, Noder M, Riederer P (1989) Effects of glucocorticoids on plasma catecholamines in depression. Psychiatry Res 29(2):187–198

85. Rydmark I, Wahlberg K, Ghatan PH, Modell S, Nygren A, Ingvar M, Asberg M, Heilig M (2006) Neuroendocrine, cognitive and structural imaging characteristics of women on long-term sickleave with job stress-induced depression. Biol Psychiatry 60(8):867–873. doi:10.1016/j.biopsych.2006.04.029, S0006–3223(06)00563–4 [pii]

86. Salloway S, Correia S, Boyle P, Malloy P, Schneider L, Lavretsky H, Sackheim H, Roose S, Krishnan KRR (2002) MRI subcortical hyperintensities in old and very old depressed outpatients: The important role of age in late-life depression. Journal of the neurological sciences 203–204:227–233. doi:http://dx.doi.org/10.1016/S0022-510X(02)00296-4

87. Sassi RB, Brambilla P, Nicoletti M, Mallinger AG, Frank E, Kupfer DJ, Keshavan MS, Soares JC (2003) White matter hyperintensities in bipolar and unipolar patients with relatively mild-to-moderate illness severity. J Affect Disord 77(3):237–245

88. Serretti A, Mandelli L, Bajo E, Cevenini N, Papili P, Mori E, Bigelli M, Berardi D (2009) The socio-economical burden of schizophrenia: a simulation of cost-offset of early intervention program in Italy. Eur Psychiatry 24(1):11–16. doi:http://dx.doi.org/10.1016/j.eurpsy.2008.07.009

89. Sheline YI, Gado MH, Price JL (1998) Amygdala core nuclei volumes are decreased in recurrent major depression. Neuroreport 9(9):2023–2028

90. Sheline YI, Pieper CF, Barch DM, Welsh-Bohmer K, McKinstry RC, MacFall JR, D'Angelo G, Garcia KS, Gersing K, Wilkins C, Taylor W, Steffens DC, Krishnan RR, Doraiswamy PM (2010) Support for the vascular depression hypothesis in late-life depression: results of a 2-site, prospective, antidepressant treatment trial. Archives of General Psychiatry 67(3):277–285. doi:10.1001/archgenpsychiatry.2009.204

91. Sheline YI, Disabato BM, Hranilovich J, Morris C, D'Angelo G, Pieper C, Toffanin T, Taylor WD, MacFall JR, Wilkins C, Barch DM, Welsh-Bohmer KA, Steffens DC, Krishnan RR, Doraiswamy PM (2012) Treatment course with antidepressant therapy in late-life depression. The American Journal of Psychiatry 169(11):1185–1193

92. Sher L, Oquendo MA, Burke AK, Cooper TB, Mann JJ (2013) Combined dexamethasone suppression-corticotrophin-releasing hormone stimulation test in medication-free major depression and healthy volunteers. J Affect Disord 151(3):1108–1112. doi:10.1016/j.jad.2013.06.049, S0165–0327(13)00529–6 [pii]

93. Smith R, Chen K, Baxter L, Fort C, Lane RD (2013) Antidepressant effects of sertraline associated with volume increases in dorsolateral prefrontal cortex. J Affect Disord 146(3):414–419. doi:http://dx.doi.org/10.1016/j.jad.2012.07.029

94. Sneed JR, Culang-Reinlieb ME, Brickman AM, Gunning-Dixon FM, Johnert L, Garcon E, Roose SP (2011) MRI signal hyperintensities and failure to remit following antidepressant treatment. Journal of affective disorders 135(1–3):315–320. doi:http://dx.doi.org/10.1016/j.jad.2011.06.052

95. Sullivan EV, Marsh L, Mathalon DH, Lim KO, Pfefferbaum A (1995) Anterior hippocampal volume deficits in nonamnesic, aging chronic alcoholics. Alcohol Clin Exp Res 19(1):110–122

96. Taylor WD, Kudra K, Zhao Z, Steffens DC, MacFall JR (2014) Cingulum bundle white matter lesions influence antidepressant response in late-life depression: a pilot study. J Affect Disord 162(0):8–11. doi:http://dx.doi.org/10.1016/j.jad.2014.03.031

97. Uher R, Huezo-Diaz P, Perroud N, Smith R, Rietschel M, Mors O, Hauser J, Maier W, Kozel D, Henigsberg N, Barreto M, Placentino A, Dernovsek MZ, Schulze TG, Kalember P, Zobel A, Czerski PM, Larsen ER, Souery D, Giovannini C, Gray JM, Lewis CM, Farmer A, Aitchison KJ, McGuffin P, Craig I (2009) Genetic predictors of response to antidepressants in the GENDEP project. Pharmacogenomics J 9(4):225–233. doi:10.1038/tpj.2009.12, tpj200912 [pii]

98. Uher R, Tansey KE, Dew T, Maier W, Mors O, Hauser J, Dernovsek MZ, Henigsberg N, Souery D, Farmer A, McGuffin P (2014) An inflammatory biomarker as a differential predictor of outcome of depression treatment with escitalopram and nortriptyline. Am J Psychiatry 171(12):1278–1286. doi:10.1176/appi.ajp.2014.14010094

99. van Eijndhoven P, van Wingen G, Katzenbauer M, Groen W, Tepest R, Fernandez G, Buitelaar J, Tendolkar I (2013) Paralimbic cortical thickness in first-episode depression: evidence for trait-related differences in mood regulation. Am J Psychiatry 170(12):1477–1486. doi:10.1176/appi.ajp.2013.12121504

100. Vakili K, Pillay SS, Lafer B, Fava M, Renshaw PF, Bonello-Cintron CM, Yurgelun-Todd DA (2000) Hippocampal volume in primary unipolar major depression: a magnetic resonance imaging study. Biological psychiatry 47(12):1087–1090. doi:10.1016/S0006-3223(99)00296-6

101. Vythilingam M, Heim C, Newport J, Miller AH, Anderson E, Bronen R, Brummer M, Staib L, Vermetten E, Charney DS, Nemeroff CB, Bremner JD (2002) Childhood trauma associated with smaller hippocampal volume in women with major depression. Am J Psychiatry 159(12):2072–2080

102. Vythilingam M, Vermetten E, Anderson GM, Luckenbaugh D, Anderson ER, Snow J, Staib LH, Charney DS, Bremner JD (2004) Hippocampal volume, memory, and cortisol status in major depressive disorder: effects of treatment. Biol Psychiatry 56(2):101–112. doi:10.1016/j.biopsych.2004.04.002

103. Warner-Schmidt JL, Vanover KE, Chen EY, Marshall JJ, Greengard P (2011) Antidepressant effects of selective serotonin reuptake inhibitors (SSRIs) are attenuated by antiinflammatory drugs in mice and humans. Proc Natl Acad Sci U S A 108(22):9262–9267. doi:10.1073/pnas.1104836108

104. Xiong P, Zeng Y, Wu Q, Han Huang DX, Zainal H, Xu X, Wan J, Xu F, Lu J (2014) Combining serum protein concentrations to diagnose schizophrenia: a preliminary exploration. J Clin Psychiatry 75(8):e794–e801. doi:10.4088/JCP.13m0877

105. Yuen GS, Gunning FM, Woods E, Klimstra SA, Hoptman MJ, Alexopoulos GS (2014) Neuroanatomical correlates of apathy in late-life depression and antidepressant treatment response. J Affect Disord 166(0):179–186. doi:http://dx.doi.org/10.1016/j.jad.2014.05.008

Chapter 6
Pharmacogenetics of Mood Stabilizers

Janusz K. Rybakowski

Abstract Mood stabilizers form a cornerstone in the long-term treatment of bipolar disorder (BD). Along with carbamazepine and valproates, lithium belongs to the first generation of mood stabilizers which appeared in psychiatric treatment in the 1960s. Atypical antipsychotics with mood-stabilizing properties and lamotrigine which were introduced in the mid-1990s form the second generation of such drugs. The main phenotype of the response to mood stabilizers is a degree of prevention against recurrences of manic and depressive episodes during long-term treatment. The vast majority of data on genetic influences on the response to mood stabilizers has been gathered in relation to lithium. The studies on the mechanisms of lithium action and on the neurobiology of bipolar disorder have led to the identification of a number of candidate genes connected with neurotransmitters, second messengers, neuroprotection, circadian rhythms, pathogenesis of BD, and those located on chromosome 22q11–13. There are few published pharmacogenomic studies of other mood stabilizers than lithium, mostly on valproate. In recent years, a number of genome-wide association studies (GWAS) in bipolar disorders have been performed, and some of those have also focused on lithium response. Recently, the first data appeared from the Consortium on Lithium Genetics (ConLiGen) establishing the largest sample, to date, for the GWAS of lithium response in bipolar disorder. The study of 2563 patients collected by 22 participating sites demonstrated an association between lithium response and two long noncoding RNAs located on chromosome 21.

6.1 Introduction

Mood stabilizers form a cornerstone in the long-term treatment of bipolar disorder, which is a serious mental illness, with a worldwide prevalence of 2–5 % of the population [42]. A mood stabilizer can be defined as a drug that if used

J.K. Rybakowski
Department of Adult Psychiatry, Poznan University of Medical Sciences,
ul.Szpitalna 27/33, Poznan 60-572, Poland
e-mail: janusz.rybakowski@gmail.com

© Springer International Publishing Switzerland 2016   93
J.K. Rybakowski, A. Serretti (eds.), *Genetic Influences on Response to Drug Treatment for Major Psychiatric Disorders*, DOI 10.1007/978-3-319-27040-1_6

as monotherapy (1) acts therapeutically in mania and/or in depression; (2) acts prophylactically against manic and/or depressive episodes, as demonstrated in a trial of at least 1 year's duration; and (3) does not worsen any therapeutic or prophylactic aspect of the illness outlined above. Several years ago, a classification of mood stabilizers based on the chronology of their introduction for the treatment of bipolar mood disorder has been proposed by the author of this chapter [53].

The first generation of mood stabilizers began to be introduced more than half a century ago, with lithium being the earliest drug of this kind [17], followed by anticonvulsants such as valproates [29] and carbamazepine [45]. In the mid-1990s, American researchers suggested that the atypical antipsychotic drug, clozapine, may possess a mood-stabilizing property [93]. At the turn of twenty-first century, mood-stabilizing activity has been revealed for such atypical antipsychotics as olanzapine, quetiapine, aripiprazole, and risperidone [51, 53, 54]. A suggestion that lamotrigine is a mood-stabilizing drug was made in the early 2000s [26]. A time lag between the introduction of these two groups of mood stabilizers amounted to more than 20 years. Therefore, it has been proposed to name lithium, carbamazepine, and valproate first-generation mood stabilizers and atypical neuroleptics and lamotrigine second-generation mood stabilizers [53].

The main phenotype of response to mood stabilizers is a degree of prevention against recurrences of manic and depressive episodes during long-term treatment. Establishing the degree of response to a mood stabilizer in individual patient requires a relatively long period of follow-up. So far, the most prolonged observations were made with lithium, and so-called excellent lithium responders (not having recurrences throughout the period of lithium treatment) may constitute a genetically distinct phenotype which could be used in pharmacogenetic studies [15]. The "excellent lithium responders" constitute about 1/3 of lithium-treated bipolar patients [57]. The effect of lithium maintenance treatment can be assessed either retrospectively or prospectively and the response can be expressed in either categorical or dimensional terms. Although the duration of treatment with mood stabilizers other than lithium is much shorter, such assessment can be also adapted to anticonvulsants and atypical antipsychotics having mood-stabilizing properties.

The lithium-treated patients in the Department of Adult Psychiatry, Poznan University of Medical Sciences who were involved in our pharmacogenetic studies had a duration of lithium prophylaxis of at least 5 years (5–27, mean 15 years) allowing us to retrospectively assess the degree of lithium response accurately. In our studies, excellent lithium responders were contrasted with patients showing only a partial response, i.e., a 50 % reduction in the episode index (number of episodes per year, compared to the pre-lithium period) and with those showing no response (>50 % reduction, no change or a worsening in the episode index) [58]. In the majority of other papers, the response to lithium has also been assessed retrospectively, although the criteria for response have been defined in various ways. Usually, two categories of patients (responders and nonresponders) are compared. In some papers, the response to lithium has been established prospectively, by comparing patients in whom recurrence occurred within a period of prospective observation (usually 2–3 years) with those without such a recurrence [73].

In 2002, the Canadian researchers introduced a scale allowing quantitative retrospective assessment of the quality of prophylactic lithium response [14]. This scale is referred to as "the Alda scale" since one of the team's member, Martin Alda, was most instrumental for its development. In this scale, criterion A rates the degree of response (activity of the illness while on adequate lithium treatment) on a ten-point scale. Criteria B1–B5 establish whether there is a causal relationship between the improvement and the treatment. Criterion B involves B1: the number of episodes off the treatment, B2: frequency of episode off the treatment, B3: the duration of treatment, B4: compliance during period(s) of stability, and B5: the use of additional medications during the periods of stability. The total score is obtained by subtracting B from A and is in the range 0–10. Therefore, this scale allows for either a categorical assessment (i.e., below or above some cutoff point) or a dimensional assessment of lithium response. It has therefore been used in the Consortium of Lithium Genetics (ConLiGen) project aimed at performing a genome-wide association study (GWAS) in a large population of lithium-treated patients. The results of assessments including 29 ConLiGen sites covering 1308 patients showed substantial and moderate agreement across sites, with two definitions of lithium response, one dichotomous and the other continuous [36].

A number of reviews on the pharmacogenetics of mood stabilizers in bipolar disorder were published in recent years, the most important including those by Rybakowski [55], Severino et al. [76], and Geoffroy et al. [13]. They were mostly focused on the candidate genes with little mentioning of the genome-wide association studies (GWAS). In this chapter, the numerous candidate genes connected with lithium and other mood stabilizers will be reviewed, followed by the results of the GWAS studies, focused mostly on lithium, including also the first results of the ConLiGen project (Tables 6.1 and 6.2).

6.2 Linkage Studies of Lithium Response

Prior to candidate gene studies, there had been some linkage studies of susceptibility loci specifically analyzing those connected with lithium response. Danish investigators [12] performed a haplotype-based study in lithium-responding patients with bipolar disorder on the Faroe Islands and found chromosomal region 18q23 to possibly be connected with lithium response. Canadian researchers [89] after having performed a genome scan of 31 families ascertained, through probands with an excellent lithium response, that the locus on chromosome 7q11 may be implicated. However, in spite of the susceptibility regions found in these studies, no specific genes have been identified (Table 6.2).

Table 6.1 Pharmacogenetics of mood stabilizers: candidate gene studies

Mood stabilizer	Neurobiology area	Positive findings	Authors
Lithium	Neurotransmission	5-HTT gene TPH gene DRD1 gene FYN gene	Serretti et al. [72, 74], Rybakowski et al. [59], Tharoor et al. [87] Serretti et al. [69] Rybakowski et al. [61] Szczepankiewicz et al. [83]
	Intracellular second messengers	INPP1 gene CREB1 gene	Steen et al. [81] Mamdani et al. [32]
	Neuroprotection	BDNF gene NTRK2 gene GSK3β gene miRNA Let-7 gene	Rybakowski et al. [58] Dmitrzak-Weglarz et al. [10] Leckband et al. [30] Benedetti et al. [2] Hunsberger et al. [22]
	Circadian rhythms	Rev-Erbα gene ARNTL gene TIM gene DPB gene	Campos-de-Souza et al. [4], McCarthy et al. [40] Rybakowski et al. [64] Rybakowski et al. [64] Kittel-Schneider et al. [28]
	Pathogenesis of bipolar disorder	NR3C1 gene DISC-1 gene mDNA	Szczepankiewicz et al. [86] Czerski et al. [7] Washizuka et al. [91]
	Chromosome 22q11–13	BCR gene XBP1 gene CACNG2 gene	Masui et al. [39] Masui et al. [37, 38] Silberberg et al. [77]
Valproate	Chromosome 22q11–13	XBP1 gene	Kim et al. [27]

Positive findings for association of prophylactic response with candidate genes
Abbreviations: *5-HTT* serotonin transporter. *TRH* tryptophan hydroxylase, *DRD1* dopamine receptor 1, *FYN* tyrosine kinase fyn, *INPP1* inositol polyphosphate 1-phosphatase, *CREB1* cAMP response element-binding protein 1, *BDNF* brain-derived neurotrophic factor, *GSK3β* glycogen synthase kinase beta, *miRNA* microRNA, *ARNTL* aryl hydrocarbon receptor nuclear translocator-like, *TIM* timeless clock, *DPG* albumin D-box binding protein, *NR3C1* glucocorticoid receptor, *DISC-1* Disrupted-in-Schizophrenia 1, *BCR* breakpoint cluster region, *XBP1* X-box binding protein, *CACNG2* calcium channel gamma-2 subunit

6.3 Candidate Gene Studies of Lithium Response

6.3.1 Neurotransmitters

The serotonergic system has long been implicated in the neurobiology of bipolar disorder and the mechanism of lithium action [44]. For pharmacogenetic studies, a subject of special interest has been a functional promoter polymorphism of the serotonin transporter gene (5-HTTLPR) located on chromosome 17q12 where a short (s) allele is connected with lower activity of the gene. A short allele of 5-HTTLPR has been associated with a predisposition to affective disorder, both bipolar and unipolar [19] and with a poor response to antidepressants in a Caucasian population

Table 6.2 Pharmacogenetics of lithium: linkage and GWAS studies

Type of study	Positive finding	Authors
Linkage study: lithium responders on the Faroe Islands Linkage study: Canadian families of lithium responders)	Region 18q23 Region 7q11	Ewald et al. [12] Turecki et al. [89]
GWAS: family-based association study of BD patients for lithium-related genes GWAS: data from STEP-BD study GWAS: lithium-treated Sardinian patients GWAS: ConLiGen GWAS: lymphoblastoid cells from lithium-treated patients GWAS: Taiwan Bipolar Consortium GWAS: ConLiGen	None Regions 3p2, 28q22, 11q14, 15q26; *GRIA2* gene *ACCN1* gene *SCL4A10* gene *IGF-1* gene *GADL1* gene 2 lncRNAs on chromosome 21	Perlis et al. [47] Perlis et al. [48] Squassina et al. [79] Schulze [65] Squassina et al. [80] Chen et al. [5] Hou et al. [21]

Positive findings of linkage and genome-wide association studies (GWAS)

Abbreviations: *STEP-BD* systematic treatment enhancement program for bipolar disorder, *ConLiGen* consortium on lithium genetics, *GRIA2* glutamate AMPA receptor 1, *ACCN1* amiloride-sensitive cation channel 1 neuronal, *SCL4A10* solute carrier family 4, sodium bicarbonate transporter, member 10, *IGF-1* insulin-like growth factor-1, *GADL1* glutamate decarboxylase-like protein 1, *lncRNA* long noncoding RNA

[50]. That the s allele may be connected with prophylactic lithium nonresponse was demonstrated in several studies, including ours [59, 72, 74] but was not confirmed in two subsequent papers [34, 43]. Recently, Tharoor et al. [87] studied the serotonin transporter triallelic 5-HTTLPR and intron 2 (STin2) polymorphisms in relation to lithium response in Indian population and found a possible association with STin2 and a combined effect with 5-HTTLPR variants suggesting better efficacy of lithium in patients carrying 5-HTT polymorphisms associated with reduced transcriptional activity.

Studies on an association between lithium response and the genes of the serotonergic receptors 5-HT1, 5-HT2A, and 5-HT2C yielded negative results [9, 71]. On the other hand, one study on a polymorphism on the gene for tryptophan hydroxylase, the enzyme of serotonin synthesis, found a marginal association [69].

Severino et al. [75] showed an association between bipolar illness and A48G polymorphism of the dopaminergic receptor D1 (DRD1) gene located on chromosome 5q35, and we have demonstrated an association of this polymorphism with lithium response [61]. Earlier studies on other dopaminergic system genes (DRD2, DRD3, DRD4) brought negative results [68, 70]. Also negative were the results of studies on an association between lithium response and polymorphisms of genes coding enzymes of catecholamine metabolism such as monoamine oxidase (MAO) and catechol-O-methyltransferase (COMT) [73, 88].

The glutamatergic system has been recently implicated in the pathogenesis of bipolar illness and the mechanisms of lithium action, with special emphasis on such glutamate receptors as NMDA (N-methyl-D-aspartate) and AMPA (alpha-amino-3-hydroxy-5 methyl-4-isoxazolepropionate). In our study we did not demonstrate any association between three polymorphisms in the NMDA receptor 2B subunit

(*GRIN2B*) gene and lithium response [83]. On the other hand, our group showed an association between two polymorphisms of the FYN gene and bipolar disorder [84] and a marginal association between T/C polymorphism of this gene and lithium response [85]. The Src family, tyrosine kinase FYN, plays a key role in the interaction between the glutamatergic receptor NMDA and the brain-derived neurotrophic factor (BDNF), and the *FYN* gene is located on chromosome 6q21, the susceptibility region for bipolar disorder.

6.3.2 Intracellular Second Messengers

The effect on the phosphatidylinositol (PI) pathway has long been considered the most important mechanism of lithium therapeutic action in bipolar disorder. A significant association with lithium response was obtained with polymorphism of the inositol polyphosphate 1-phosphatase (*INPP1*) gene located on chromosome 2q32 [81]. Such an association with lithium response was also obtained in bipolar patients with comorbid post-traumatic stress disorder [3], but this was not replicated in a study by Brazilian investigators [43]. Studies on the polymorphisms of other genes connected with the PI system, such as inositol monophosphatase2 (*IMPA2*) and diacylglycerol kinase eta (*DGKH*) genes, did not find any associations with lithium response [8, 35].

Lithium also exerts an effect on the cyclic adenosine monophosphate (cAMP) pathway. Mamdani et al. [32] performed an association study with genes for cAMP response element-binding protein (CREB) and found an association between bipolar disorder and lithium response and two polymorphisms of *CREB1* gene located at chromosome 2q32–34.

Lithium interacts with the protein kinase C (PKC) pathway, a mediator of intracellular responses to neurotransmitter signaling, and PDLIM5 is an adaptor protein that selectively binds the isozyme PKC epsilon to N-type calcium channels in neurons. Squassina et al. [78] did not find an association between the *PDLIM5* gene polymorphisms and lithium response.

6.3.3 Substances Involved in Neuroprotection

BDNF is a neurotrophic factor involved in neuronal proliferation and synaptic plasticity. Lithium has been shown to stimulate the BDNF system both in experimental and clinical conditions that makes one of the main mechanisms of lithium's neuroprotective activity [52]. An association of Val66Met functional polymorphism of the *BDNF* gene, located on chromosome 11p13, with bipolar disorder has been suggested [67], and our group was the first to demonstrate an association of this polymorphism with lithium response [10, 58]. Furthermore, we have found a significant interaction of this polymorphism with that of the serotonin transporter where, in subjects with the s allele of 5-HTTLPR having a Val/Val genotype of BDNF, there is a 70 % probability of lithium nonresponse [60]. However, an association of lithium response with Val66Met polymorphism of the *BDNF* gene was not confirmed in populations other than Caucasian [37, 43]. The neurotrophin BDNF binds to the TrkB receptor, transcribed from the *NTRK2* gene. The San Diego group of investigators has suggested an association of this polymorphism with lithium response in bipolar patients with higher suicidality and euphoric mania [30]; however, we were not able to find such an association in our sample of bipolar patients [10].

Lithium inhibits glycogen synthase kinase 3 beta (GSK3β), the enzyme involved in synaptic plasticity, apoptosis, and the circadian cycle. Italian investigators demonstrated an association between functional −50 T/C polymorphism of the *GSK3β* gene located on chromosome 3q13 and lithium response [2], but this was not confirmed in two other studies, including ours [43, 82].

Recently, a novel integrative genomic tool called GRANITE (Genetic Regulatory Analysis of Networks Investigational Tool Environment) for analyzing large complex genetic data has been developed. In an in vitro study comparing vehicle versus chronic lithium treatment in lymphoblastoid cells derived from either lithium responders or nonresponders, it was found that the microRNAs (miRNAs) of Let-7 family were downregulated in both lithium groups. This miRNA family has been implicated in neurodegeneration, cell survival, and synaptic development [22].

6.3.4   The Circadian Signaling System

Lithium has been shown to influence circadian processes. As mentioned above, GSK3β, the enzyme inhibited by lithium, is also involved in regulation of circadian cycle. In a network coordinating circadian rhythms, GSK3β interacts with a number of proteins including nuclear receptor rev-erb alpha (Rev- Erb-α). A variant of *Rev-Erb-α* gene has been shown, in two studies, to be associated with prophylactic lithium response [4, 40].

In our study of lithium-treated bipolar patients, we genotyped single nucleotide polymorphisms (SNPs) and haplotypes of four circadian clock genes in relation to prophylactic lithium response. The genes included *CLOCK* (circadian locomotor output cycle kaput), *ARNTL* (aryl hydrocarbon receptor nuclear translocator-like), *TIM* (timeless circadian clock), and *PER 3* (period circadian clock-3). An association with the degree of lithium prophylaxis was found for six SNPs and three haplotype blocks of the *ARNTL* gene and two SNPs and on haplotype block of the *TIM* gene, while no association with SNPs or haplotypes of the *CLOCK* and *PER-3* genes was observed [64].

Recently, Kittel-Schneider et al. [28] in a study of lymphoblastoid cells generated from bipolar patients and control subjects demonstrated that these two groups differed in the length period regarding expression of another clock gene, namely, *DBP* (albumin D-box binding protein) gene, and that chronic lithium treatment leads to decreased expression of this gene.

6.3.5   Genes Associated with Pathogenesis of BD

Our group found an association of prophylactic lithium response in bipolar patients with polymorphism of two genes implicated in the pathogenesis of bipolar disorder, namely, the glucocorticoid receptor (*NR3C1*) gene located on chromosome 5q31–32 [86] and the Disrupted-in-Schizophrenia (*DISC-1*) gene located on chromosome 1q42 [7]. Also, Japanese researchers in considering postulated abnormalities of mitochondrial DNA (mDNA) in bipolar disorder [25] demonstrated an association between 10398A mDNA polymorphism and the quality of lithium prophylaxis [91].

Matrix metalloproteinase-9 (MMP-9) is an extracellularly acting endopeptidase implicated in a number of pathological conditions including cancer, cardiovascular, and neuropsychiatric diseases. Our group demonstrated an association between functional polymorphism of the *MMP-9* gene, located on chromosome 20q11–13, and bipolar disorder [62]. However, we were unable to find such an association with lithium response [63]. Also, Canadian investigators studied the prolyl endopeptidase (*PREP*) gene, located on chromosome 6q22, the region that has been linked to bipolar disorder in several studies, but did not find an association with lithium response [33].

6.3.6   Genes Located on 22q11–13

Positive results with lithium response have been obtained concerning associations of three genes located on chromosome 22q11–13, a possible susceptibility region for major psychoses. Japanese authors found a significant association between lithium response and genetic variations in the breakpoint cluster region (*BCR*) gene located on chromosome 22q11 [39] and with the X-box binding protein 1 (*XBP1*) gene located on chromosome 22q12 [38]. An association of both these genes with a predisposition to bipolar disorder had been previously reported [18, 24]. Silberberg et al. [77] described an association with lithium response and the calcium channel gamma-2 subunit (*CACNG2*) gene, also known as stargazin, located on chromosome 22q13.

6.4   Studies on Candidate Genes of Response to Other Mood Stabilizers

Only few studies have focused on the candidate genes of response to other mood stabilizers, mostly to valproate. Korean researchers studied functional –116C/G polymorphism of the XBP1 gene in relation to valproate efficacy [27]. Interestingly, they found an association with a positive prophylactic effect for valproate with the C allele of this polymorphism, while with lithium it was with the G allele [37, 38].

This may suggest that the response to different mood stabilizers may be connected with a different genetic makeup.

There are other studies which are of short duration and do not differentiate between individual mood stabilizers (lithium, valproate, or carbamazepine). In one of them, Yun et al. [92] did not find an association between antimanic efficacy of mood stabilizers and the dysbindin (*DTNBP1*) gene variants. In another, a significant association was found between polymorphism of the *NTRK2* gene and treatment response to lithium or valproate [90]. Finally, in Lee et al. [31] study, an association was observed between the polymorphism of dopaminergic D2 receptor (DRD2/ANKK1 TaqIA) gene and treatment response in mania when dextromethorphan was added to valproate compared to adding placebo [31].

Perlis et al. [49] evaluated common genetic variations for association with symptomatic improvement in bipolar I depression following 7-week treatment with olanzapine/fluoxetine combination (OFC) or lamotrigine. They found that SNPs within the dopamine D(3) receptor and histamine H(1) receptor (HRH1) genes were significantly associated with response to OFC, while SNPs within the dopamine D(2) receptor, HRH1, dopamine beta-hydroxylase, glucocorticoid receptor, and melanocortin 2 receptor genes were significantly associated with response to lamotrigine.

6.5   Limitations of Candidate Gene Studies

Candidate gene studies have yielded a number of associations between the polymorphisms of several dozen genes and a prophylactic response to mood stabilizers, mostly lithium. However, only a minority of them has been consistently replicated in subsequent studies. Concerning lithium, each of the single nucleotide polymorphisms of a given gene accounts for a small portion of the total variance in lithium response (1–2 % at best). Therefore, lithium response is apparently polygenic and only by simultaneously examining multiple genes and multiple variants within these genes would it be possible to provide some guidelines for predicting the response. This may also apply to other mood stabilizers.

6.6   Genome-Wide Association Studies (GWAS) Focusing on Lithium Response

Perlis et al. [47] carried out a family-based association study of lithium-related and other candidate genes in bipolar disorders. Lithium genes were selected as related primarily to inositol 1,4,5-triphosphate (17 genes), to GSK3beta/Wnt signaling (39 genes), and to those implicated by messenger RNA expression data and related approaches (35 genes). Although some promising genes thought to be connected with bipolar disorder were postulated, no association with bipolar disorder was found in relation to genes specifically connected with lithium mechanisms. However, about the same time a paper appeared describing the results of GWAS in bipolar disorder, where the highest signal was obtained with the *DGKH* gene, which encodes a key protein in the lithium-sensitive phosphatidylinositol pathway [1].

In another study, Perlis et al. [48] utilized GWAS data, obtained from the Systematic Treatment Enhancement Program for Bipolar Disorder (STEP-BD) study, to examine association with risk for recurrence among patients treated with lithium and subsequently examined the regions that showed the greatest evidence of association in a second cohort of bipolar patients drawn from a clinical population at University College London. A phenotype definition was that of achieving euthymia for at least 8 weeks during prospective follow-up. It turned out that of the regions with a p value of $<5 \times 10^{-4}$ in the STEP-BD cohort, five (8q22, 3p22, 11q14, 4q32, 15q26) showed consistent evidence of association in a second cohort. The authors found a region of special interest on chromosome 4q32 spanning a *GRIA2* gene, coding for the glutamate AMPA receptor [48].

Squassina et al. [79] performed a GWAS study on lithium-treated Sardinian patients with bipolar disorder. A phenotypic assessment of lithium response was made, using the retrospective criteria of a long-term treatment response scale. The strongest association, also supported by the quantitative trait analysis, was shown for a SNP of the amiloride-sensitive cation channel 1 neuronal (*ACCN1*) gene, located on chromosome 17q12, encoding a cation channel with high affinity for sodium, and permeable to lithium. In another study, Squassina et al. [80] carried out a genome-wide expression analysis on lymphoblastoid cell lines from bipolar patients, responders, and nonresponders to lithium. It was observed that only insulin-like growth factor 1 (*IGF-1*) gene was significantly overexpressed in lithium responders compared to lithium nonresponders or healthy control subjects.

McCarthy et al. [41] analyzed GWAS studies performed in bipolar disorder, comparing the rates of genetic associations of circadian clock genes in bipolar disorder and control subjects in relation to possible lithium responsive genes, using a multi-level approach. They suggest that, despite the negative data obtained so far in GWAS, further studies on possible associations between clock genes, bipolar disorder, and lithium response are warranted.

Recently, the results of the GWAS performed by the Taiwan Bipolar Consortium, including a sample of 1761 patients of Han Chinese descent, were published. The strongest association with lithium response was obtained for two SNPs of glutamate decarboxylase-like protein 1 (*GADL1*) gene located at chromosome 3p24.1 [5]. However, subsequent studies performed by other groups failed to replicate these findings in either Asian or European ancestry samples [6, 20, 23].

It should be also mentioned that another prospective, multicenter trial named Pharmacogenomics of Mood Stabilizer Response in Bipolar Disorder (PGBD) with John Kelsoe as a principal investigator is underway where lithium is an important part. An abstract describing the study is available on the web: http://pgrn.org/display/pgrnwevsite/PGBD+Profile

6.7   Consortium on Lithium Genetics (ConLiGen)

Following an initiative by the International Group for the Study of Lithium-Treated Patient and the Unit on the Genetic Basis of Mood and Anxiety Disorders at the National Institute of Mental Health, lithium researchers from around the world have formed the Consortium on Lithium Genetics (ConLiGen) in order to establish the largest sample to date for genome-wide studies of lithium response in bipolar disorder [66].

The first results of the ConLiGen initiative were presented during a CINP meeting in Stockholm in 2012. The GWAS top hit ($p = 1.52 \times 10^{-6}$) was found for the *SLC4A10* gene coding solute carrier family 4, sodium bicarbonate transporter, member 10, which belongs to a family of sodium-coupled bicarbonate transporters [65]. This gene is located on chromosome 2q24 and is highly expressed in the hippocampus and cerebral cortex. It has been implicated in complex partial epilepsy and mental retardation [16]. The bicarbonate sensitive pathway is the most important mechanism for active lithium influx into the cell [11]. However, these results have not been replicated in a different sample.

Recently, the results of the ConLiGen GWAS, including 2563 patients collected by 22 participating sites, were reported. Data from over 6 million common SNPs were tested for association with both categorical and continuous rating of lithium response. The response-associated region on chromosome 21, containing two long noncoding RNAs (lncRNAs), was identified [21]. Although noncoding, the lcnRNA have been increasingly appreciated as important regulators of gene expression, particularly in the central nervous system. However, the biological context of these findings and their clinical utility remains to be further elucidated.

6.8   Conclusions

The pharmacogenetics of response to mood stabilizers has recently become a growing field of research, especially in relation to the pharmacogenetics of lithium prophylaxis of bipolar disorder but also to other mood-stabilizing drugs. Candidate gene studies revealed nearly hundred genes that may be associated with the prophylactic efficacy of such drugs in BD. However, considering obvious limitations of candidate gene studies such as low statistical power or only few or even a single marker per gene studied, the GWAS studies and, especially, the ConLiGen project make an important step forward in this research. Future studies will need to focus on replication of the GWAS findings in independent samples (Table 6.2).

Possible practical implications of these pharmacogenetic studies have yet to be seen. It may be assumed that the response to any mood stabilizer is connected with the interaction of multiple genes, as demonstrated in relation to lithium response. It may be supposed that the genetic makeup for response to mood stabilizers other than lithium may be different and probably specific to each drug. Furthermore, the genes for response to a mood stabilizer may be dependent on the peculiarity of the clinical picture of BD. The clinical profile of lithium-responding BD patients was recently proposed [56], and some attempts for such a profile were also made for lamotrigine [46]. Therefore, there is increasing hope that clinicians will eventually be assisted by a panel of genetic tests that, according to the assumptions of personalized medicine, may successfully predict which individual bipolar disorder patient is the most likely to respond to lithium or to other mood stabilizers.

References

1. Baum AE, Akula N, Cabanero M, Cardona I, Corona W, Klemens B et al (2008) A genome-wide association study implicates diacylglycerol kinase eta (DGKH) and several other genes in the etiology of bipolar disorder. Mol Psychiatry 13:197–207
2. Benedetti F, Serretti A, Pontigia A, Bernasconi A, Lorenzi C, Colombo C et al (2005) Long-term response to lithium salts in bipolar illness is influenced by the glycogen synthase kinase 3-beta- 50T/C SNP. Neurosci Lett 376:51–55
3. Bremer T, Diamond C, McKinney R, Shehktman T, Barrett TB, Herold C et al (2007) The pharmacogenetics of lithium response depends upon clinical co-morbidity. Mol Diagn Ther 11:161–170
4. Campos-de-Sousa S, Guindalini C, Tondo L, Munro J, Osborne S, Floris G et al (2010) Nuclear receptor rev-erb-(alpha) circadian gene variants and lithium carbonate prophylaxis in bipolar affective disorder. J Biol Rhythms 25:132–137
5. Chen CH, Lee CS, Lee MT, Ouyang WC, Chen CG, Chong MY et al (2014) Variant GADL1 and response to lithium therapy in bipolar disorder. N Engl J Med 370:119–128
6. Cruceanu C, Alda M, Dion PA, Turecki G, Rouleau GA (2015) No evidence for GADL1 variation as a bipolar disorder susceptibility factor in a Caucasian lithium-responsive cohort. Am J Psychiatry 172:94–95
7. Czerski PM, Kliwicki S, Maciukiewicz M, Hauser J, Karlowski W, Cichon S et al (2011) Multiple single nucleotide polymorphisms of schizophrenia-related DISC1 gene in lithium-treated patients with bipolar affective disorder. Eur Neuropsychopharmacol 21(Suppl 1):S4–S5
8. Dimitrova A, Milanova V, Krastev S, Nikolov I, Toncheva D, Owen MJ et al (2005) Association study of myo-inositol monophosphatase 2 (IMPA2) polymorphisms with bipolar affective disorder and response to lithium treatment. Pharmacogenomics J 5:35–41
9. Dmitrzak-Weglarz M, Rybakowski JK, Suwalska A, Słopień A, Czerski PM, Leszczyńska-Rodziewicz A et al (2005) Association studies of 5-HT2A and 5-HT2C serotonin receptor gene polymorphisms with prophylactic lithium response in bipolar patients. Pharmacol Rep 57:761–765
10. Dmitrzak-Weglarz M, Rybakowski JK, Suwalska A, Skibinska M, Leszczynska-Rodziewicz A, Szczepankiewicz A et al (2008) Association studies of the BDNF and the NTRK2 gene polymorphisms with prophylactic lithium response in bipolar patients. Pharmacogenomics 9:1595–1603
11. Ehrlich BE, Diamond JM (1979) Lithium fluxes in human erythrocytes. Am J Physiol 237:102–110
12. Ewald H, Wang AG, Vang M, Mors O, Nyegaard M, Kruse TA (1999) A haplotype-based study of lithium responding patients with bipolar affective disorder on the Faroe Islands. Psychiatr Genet 9:23–34

13. Geoffroy PA, Bellivier F, Leboyer M, Etain B (2014) Can the response to mood stabilizer be predicted in bipolar disorder? Front Biosci 6:120–138

14. Grof P, Duffy A, Cavazzoni P, Grof E, Garnham J, MacDougall M et al (2002) Is response to prophylactic lithium a familial trait? J Clin Psychiatry 63:942–947

15. Grof P (1999) Excellent lithium responders: people whose lives have been changed by lithium prophylaxis. In: Birch NJ, Gallicchio VS, Becker RW (eds) Lithium: 50 years of psychopharmacology. New Perspectives in Biomedical and Clinical Research. Weidner Publishing Group, Cheshire/Connecticut, pp 36–51

16. Gurnett CA, Veile R, Zempel J, Blackburn L, Lovett M, Bowcock A (2008) Disruption of sodium bicarbonate transporter ASLC4A10 in a patient with complex partial epilepsy and mental retardation. Arch Neurol 65:550–553

17. Hartigan G (1963) The use of lithium salts in affective disorders. Br J Psychiatry 109:810–814

18. Hashimoto R, Okada T, Kato T, Kosuga A, Tatsumi M, Kamijima K et al (2005) The breakpoint cluster region gene on chromosome 22q11 is associated with bipolar disorder. Biol Psychiatry 57:1097–1102

19. Hauser J, Leszczynska A, Samochowiec J, Czerski PM, Ostapowicz A, Chlopocka M et al (2003) Association analysis of the insertion/deletion polymorphism in serotonin transporter gene in patients with affective disorder. Eur Psychiatry 18:129–132

20. Hou L, Heilbronner U, Rietschel M, Kato T, Kuo P-H, McMahon FJ et al (2014) Variant GADL1 and response to lithium in bipolar I disorder. N Eng J Med 370:1857–1859

21. Hou L, Heilbronner U, Degenhardt F, Adli M, Akiyama K, Akula N et al (2016) Common genetic markers for lithium response in bipolar disorders. Lancet, 21 January online

22. Hunsberger JG, Chibane FL, Elkahloun AG, Henderson R, Singh R, Lawson J et al (2015) Novel integrative genomic tool for interrogating lithium response in bipolar disorder. Tansl Psychiatry 5:e504

23. Ikeda M, Kondo K, Iwata N (2014) Variant GADL1 and response to lithium in bipolar I disorder. N Eng J Med 370:1856–1857

24. Kakiuchi C, Iwamoto K, Ishiwata M, Bundo M, Kasahara T, Kusumi I et al (2003) Impaired feedback regulation of XBP1 as a genetic risk factor for bipolar disorder. Nat Genet 35:171–175

25. Kato T, Kunugi H, Nanko S, Kato N (2001) Mitochondrial DNA polymorphism in bipolar disorder. J Affect Disord 62:151–164

26. Ketter T, Calabrese JR (2002) Stabilization of mood from below versus above baseline in bipolar disorder: a new nomenclature. J Clin Psychiatry 63:146–151

27. Kim B, Kim CY, Lee MJ, Joo YH (2009) Preliminary evidence on the association between XBP1-116C/G polymorphism and response to prophylactic treatment with valproate in bipolar disorders. Psychiatry Res 168:209–212

28. Kittel-Schneider S, Schreck S, Ziegler C, Weißflog L, Hilscher M, Schwarz R et al (2015) Lithium-induced clock gene expression in lymphoblastoid cells of bipolar affective patients. Pharmacopsychiatry 48:145–149

29. Lambert PA, Borselli S, Marcou G, Bouchardy M, Cabrol G (1971) Action thymoregulatrice a long terme de Depamide dans la psychose maniaco-depressive. Ann Med Psychol 2:442–447

30. Leckband SG, DeModena A, McKinney R, Shekhrman T, Kelsoe JR (2010) Lithium response is associated with the NTRK2 gene in a prospective study. Presented at 17th Annual Molecular Psychiatry Conference. Park City

31. Lee SY, Chen SL, Chang YH, Chen SH, Chu CH, Huang SY et al (2012) The DRD2/ANKK1 gene is associated with response to add-on dextromethorphan treatment in bipolar disorder. J Affect Disord 138:295–300

32. Mamdani F, Alda M, Grof P et al (2008) Lithium response and genetic variation in the CREB family of genes. Am J Med Genet B Neuropsychiatr Genet 147B:500–504

33. Mamdani F, Sequeira A, Alda M, Grof P, Rouleau G, Turecki G (2007) No association between the PREP gene and lithium responsive bipolar disorder. BMC Psychiatry 7:9

34. Manchia M, Congiu D, Squassina A, Lampus S, Ardau R, Chillotti C et al (2009) No association between lithium full responders and the DRD1, DRD2, DRD3, DAT1, 5-HTTLPR and HTR2A genes in a Sardinian sample. Psychiatry Res 169:164–166

35. Manchia M, Squassina A, Congiu D, Chillotti C, Ardau R, Severino G et al (2009) Interacting genes in lithium prophylaxis: preliminary results of an exploratory analysis on the role of DGKH and NR1D1 gene polymorphisms in 199 Sardinian bipolar patients. Neurosci Lett 467:67–71

36. Manchia M, Adli M, Akula N, Ardau R, Aubry JM, Backlund L et al (2013) Assessment of response to lithium maintenance treatment in bipolar disorder: a consortium on lithium genetics (ConLiGen) report. PLoS One 8:e65636

37. Masui T, Hashimoto R, Kusumi I, Suzuki K, Tanaka T, Nakagawa S et al (2006) Lithium response and Val66Met polymorphism of the brain derived neurotrophic factor gene in Japanese patients with bipolar disorder. Psychiatr Genet 16:49–50

38. Masui T, Hashimoto R, Kusumi I, Suzuki K, Tanaka T, Nakagawa S et al (2006) A possible association between the -116C/G single nucleotide polymorphism of the XBP1 gene and lithium prophylaxis in bipolar disorder. Int J Neuropsychopharmacol 9:83–88

39. Masui T, Hashimoto R, Kusumi I, Suzuki K, Tanaka T, Nakagawa S et al (2008) A possible association between missense polymorphism of the breakpoint cluster region gene and lithium prophylaxis in bipolar disorder. Prog Neuropsychopharmacol Biol Psychiatry 32:204–208

40. McCarthy MJ, Nievergelt CM, Shenkhtman T, Kripke DF, Welsh DK, Kelsoe JR (2011) Functional genetic variation in the Rev-Erbα pathway and lithium response in the treatment of bipolar disorder. Genes Brain Behav 10:852–861

41. McCarthy MJ, Nievergelt CM, Kelsoe JR, Welsh DK (2012) A survey of genomic studies supports association of circadian clock genes with bipolar disorder spectrum illnesses and lithium response. PLoS One 7:e32091

42. Merinkangas KR, Tohen M (2011) Epidemiology of bipolar disorder in adults and children. In: Tsuang MT, Tohen MT, Jones PB (eds) Textbook in psychiatric epidemiology. John Wiley and Sons, Chichester, pp 329–342

43. Michelon L, Meira-Lima I, Cordeiro Q, Miguita K, Breen G, Collier D et al (2006) Association study of the INPP1, 5HTT, BDNF, AP-2beta and GSK-3beta gene variants and retrospectively scored response to lithium prophylaxis in bipolar disorder. Neurosci Lett 403:288–293

44. Müller-Oerlinghausen B (1985) Lithium long-term treatment – does it act via serotonin? Pharmacopsychiatry 18:214–217

45. Okuma T, Kishimoto A, Inue K (1973) Anti-manic and prophylactic effect of carbamazepine (Tegretol) on manic depressive psychosis. Folia Psychiatr Neurol Japn 27:283–297

46. Passmore MJ, Garnham J, Duffy A, MacDougall M, Munro A, Slaney C et al (2003) Phenotypic spectra of bipolar disorder in responders to lithium versus lamotrigine. Bipolar Disord 5:110–114

47. Perlis RH, Purcell S, Fagerness J, Kirby A, Petryshen TL, Fan J et al (2008) Family-based association study of lithium-related and other candidate genes in bipolar disorder. Arch Gen Psychiatry 65:53–61

48. Perlis RH, Smoller JW, Ferreira MA, McQuillin A, Bass N, Lawrence J et al (2009) A genome-wide association study of response to lithium for prevention of recurrence in bipolar disorder. Am J Psychiatry 166:718–725

49. Perlis RH, Adams DH, Fijal B, Sutton VK, Farmen M, Breier A et al (2010) Genetic association study of treatment response with olanzapine/fluoxetine combination or lamotrigine in bipolar I depression. J Clin Psychiatry 71:599–605

50. Porcelli S, Fabbri C, Serretti A (2012) Meta-analysis of serotonin transporter gene promoter polymorphism (5-HTTLPR) association with antidepressant efficacy. Eur Neuropsychopharmacol 22:239–258

51. Quiroz JA, Yatham LN, Palumbo JM, Karcher K, Kushner S, Kusumakar V (2010) Risperidone long-acting injectable monotherapy in the maintenance treatment of bipolar disorder. Biol Psychiatry 68:156–162

52. Rowe MK, Chuang DM (2004) Lithium neuroprotection: molecular mechanisms and clinical implications. Expert Rev Mol Med 6:1–18
53. Rybakowski JK (2007) Two generations of mood stabilizers. Int J Neuropsychopharmacol 10:709–711
54. Rybakowski JK (2008) Aripiprazole joins the family of second-generation mood stabilizers. J Clin Psychiatry 69:862–863
55. Rybakowski JK (2013) Genetic influences on response to mood stabilizers in bipolar disorder. Current status of knowledge. CNS Drugs 27:165–173
56. Rybakowski JK (2014) Factors associated with lithium efficacy in bipolar disorder. Harv Rev Psychiatry 22:353–357
57. Rybakowski JK, Chłopocka-Woźniak M, Suwalska A (2001) The prophylactic effect of long-term lithium administration in bipolar patients entering lithium treatment in the 1970s and 1980s. Bipolar Disord 3:63–67
58. Rybakowski JK, Suwalska A, Skibinska M, Szczepankiewicz A, Leszczynska-Rodziewicz A, Permoda A et al (2005) Prophylactic lithium response and polymorphism of the brain-derived neurotrophic factor gene. Pharmacopsychiatry 38:166–170
59. Rybakowski JK, Suwalska A, Czerski PM, Dmitrzak-Weglarz M, Leszczynska-Rodziewicz A, Hauser J (2005) Prophylactic effect of lithium in bipolar affective illness may be related to serotonin transporter genotype. Pharmacol Rep 57:124–127
60. Rybakowski JK, Suwalska A, Skibinska M, Dmitrzak-Weglarz M, Leszczynska-Rodziewicz A et al (2007) Response to lithium prophylaxis: interaction between serotonin transporter and BDNF genes. Am J Med Genet B Neuropsychiatr Genet 144B:820–823
61. Rybakowski JK, Dmitrzak-Weglarz M, Suwalska A (2009) Dopamine D1 receptor gene polymorphism is associated with prophylactic lithium response in bipolar disorder. Pharmacopsychiatry 42:20–22
62. Rybakowski JK, Skibinska M, Leszczynska-Rodziewicz A, Kaczmarek L, Hauser J (2009) Matrix metalloproteinase-9 (MMP-9) gene and bipolar mood disorder. Neuromolecular Med 11:128–132
63. Rybakowski JK, Skibinska M, Suwalska A, Leszczynska-Rodziewicz A, Kaczmarek L, Hauser J (2011) Functional polymorphism of matrix mettaloproteinase-9 (MMP-9) gene and response to lithium prophylaxis in bipolar patients. Hum Psychopharmacol 26:168–171
64. Rybakowski JK, Dmitrzak-Weglarz M, Kliwicki S, Hauser J (2014) Polymorphism of circadian clock genes and prophylactic lithium response. Bipolar Disord 16:151–158
65. Schulze T (2012) The Consortium on Lithium Genetics (ConLiGen) genome-wide association studies of lithium response phenotypes in bipolar disorder. CINP Congress, Stockholm, Abstract book, p 36
66. Schulze TG, Alda M, Adli M, Akula N, Ardau R, Bui ET et al (2010) The International Consortium on Lithium Genetics (ConLiGen): an initiative by the NIMH and IGSLI to study the genetic basis of response to lithium treatment. Neuropsychobiology 62:72–78
67. Sears C, Markie D, Olds R, Fitches A (2011) Evidence of associations between bipolar disorder and the brain-derived neurotrophic factor (BDNF) gene. Bipolar Disord 13:630–637
68. Serretti A, Lilli R, Lorenzi C, Franchini L, Smeraldi E (1998) Dopamine receptor D3 gene and response to lithium prophylaxis in mood disorders. Int J Neuropsychopharmacol 1:125–129
69. Serretti A, Lilli R, Lorenzi C, Gasperini M, Smeraldi E (1999) Tryptophan hydroxylase gene and response to lithium prophylaxis in mood disorders. J Psychiatr Res 33:371–377
70. Serretti A, Lilli R, Lorenzi C, Franchini L, Di Bella D, Catalano M et al (1999) Dopamine receptor D2 and D4 genes, GABAA alpha-1 subunit genes and response to lithium prophylaxis in mood disorders. Psychiatry Res 87:7–19
71. Serretti A, Lorenzi C, Lilli R, Smeraldi E (2000) Serotonin receptor 2A, 2C, 1A genes and response to lithium prophylaxis in mood disorders. J Psychiatr Res 34:89–98
72. Serretti A, Lilli R, Mandelli L, Lorenzi C, Smeraldi E (2001) Serotonin transporter gene associated with lithium prophylaxis in mood disorders. Pharmacogenomics J 1:71–77

73. Serretti A, Lorenzi C, Lilli R, Mandelli L, Pirovano A, Smeraldi E (2002) Pharmacogenetics of lithium prophylaxis in mood disorders: analysis of COMT, MAO-A, and Gß3 variants. Am J Med Genet B Neuropsychiatr Genet 144:370–379

74. Serretti A, Malitas PN, Mandelli LLorenzi C, Ploia C, Alevizos B et al (2004) Further evidence for a possible association between serotonin transporter gene and lithium prophylaxis in mood disorders. Pharmacogenomics J 4:267–273

75. Severino G, Congiu D, Serreli C, De Lisa R, Chillotti C, Del Zompo M et al (2005) A48G polymorphism in the D1 receptor genes associated with bipolar I disorder. Am J Med Genet B Neuropsychiatr Genet 134B:37–38

76. Severino G, Squassina A, Costa M, Pisanu C, Calza S, Alda M et al (2013) Pharmacogenomics of bipolar disorder. Pharmacogenomics 14:655–674

77. Silberberg G, Levit A, Collier D, St Clair D, Munro J, Kerwin RW et al (2008) Stargazin involvement with bipolar disorder and response to lithium treatment. Pharmacogenet Genomics 18:403–412

78. Squassina A, Congiu D, Manconi F, Manchia M, Chillotti C, Lampus S et al (2008) The PDLIM5 gene and lithium prophylaxis: an association and gene expression analysis in Sardinian patients with bipolar disorder. Pharmacol Res 57:369–373

79. Squassina A, Manchia M, Borg J, Congiu D, Costa M, Georgitsi M et al (2011) Evidence for association of an ACCN1 gene variant with response to lithium treatment in Sardinian patients with bipolar disorder. Pharmacogenomics 12:1559–1569

80. Squassina A, Costa M, Congiu D, Manchia M, Angius A, Deiana V et al (2013) Insulin-like growth factor 1 (IGF-1) expression is up-regulated in lymphoblastoid cell lines of lithium responsive bipolar disorder patients. Pharmacol Res 73:1–7

81. Steen VM, Løvlie R, Osher Y, Belmaker RH, Berle JO, Gulbrandsen AK (1998) The polymorphic inositol polyphosphate 1-phosphatase gene as a candidate for pharmacogenetic prediction of lithium-responsive manic-depressive illness. Pharmacogenetics 8:259–268

82. Szczepankiewicz A, Rybakowski JK, Suwalska A, Skibinska M, Leszczynska-Rodziewicz A, Dmitrzak-Weglarz M et al (2006) Association study of the glycogen synthase kinase-3beta gene polymorphism with prophylactic lithium response in bipolar patients. World J Biol Psychiatry 7:158–161

83. Szczepankiewicz A, Skibinska M, Suwalska A, Hauser J, Rybakowski JK (2009) No association of three GRIN2B polymorphisms with lithium response in bipolar patients. Pharmacol Rep 61:448–452

84. Szczepankiewicz A, Rybakowski JK, Skibinska M, Dmitrzak-Weglarz M, Leszczynska-Rodziewicz A, Wilkosc M et al (2009) FYN kinase gene: another glutamatergic gene associated with bipolar disorder? Neuropsychobiology 59:178–183

85. Szczepankiewicz A, Skibinska M, Suwalska A, Hauser J, Rybakowski JK (2009) The association study of three FYN polymorphisms with prophylactic lithium response in bipolar patients. Hum Psychopharmacol 24:287–291

86. Szczepankiewicz A, Rybakowski JK, Suwalska A, Hauser J (2011) Glucocorticoid receptor polymorphism is associated with lithium response in bipolar patients. Neuro Endocrinol Lett 32:545–551

87. Tharoor H, Kotambail A, Jain S, Sharma PS, Satyamoorthy K (2013) Study of the association of serotonin transporter triallelic 5-HTTLPR and STin2 VNTR polymorphisms with lithium prophylactic response in bipolar disorder. Psychiatr Genet 23:77–81

88. Turecki G, Grof P, Cavazzoni P, Duffy A, Grof E, Ahrens B et al (1999) MAOA: association and linkage studies with lithium responsive bipolar disorder. Psychiatr Genet 9:13–16

89. Turecki G, Grof P, Grof E, D'Souza V, Lebuis L, Marineau C et al (2001) Mapping susceptibility genes for bipolar disorder: a pharmacogenetic approach based on excellent response to lithium. Mol Psychiatry 6:570–578

90. Wang Z, Fan J, Gao K, Li Z, Yi Z, Wang L et al (2013) Neurotrophic tyrosine kinase receptor type 2 (NTRK2) gene associated with treatment response to mood stabilizers in patients with bipolar I disorder. J Mol Neurosci 50:305–310

91. Washizuka S, Ikeda A, Kato N, Kato T (2003) Possible relationship between mitochondrial DNA polymorphisms and lithium response in bipolar disorder. Int J Neuropsychopharmacol 6:421–424
92. Yun DH, Pae CU, Drago A, Mandelli L, De Ronchi D, Patkar AA et al (2008) Effect of the dysbindin gene on antimanic agent in patients with bipolar I disorder. Psychiatry Investig 5:102–105
93. Zarate CA, Tohen M, Banov MD, Weiss MK, Cole JO (1995) Is clozapine a mood stabilizer? J Clin Psychiatry 56:108–112

Chapter 7
Practical Application of Pharmacogenetics of Antipsychotic, Antidepressant, and Mood-Stabilizing Drugs

Alessandro Serretti and Janusz K. Rybakowski

7.1 A Practical Example

At the doctor's office, after the first contact:

Doctor: "I understand from our consultation that you are suffering since some months from a major depressive episode and that you may benefit from a specific antidepressant treatment. I have to add that however the treatment will take a few weeks to exert its effect and there is a chance of about 50 % that it will not benefit you because of either lack of efficacy or poor tolerability."

Patient: "I see Doctor, do you have a suggestion for a prescription which could fit my situation?"

Doctor: "Yes, indeed, based on your disease profile and the information you provided me, I have in mind a few options, but now we have a further help coming from the knowledge of your genetic status. In fact we now can know in advance which of the possible options are better indicated for your case."

Patient: "What should I do then?"

Doctor: "If you agree, I will collect with this buccal swab a specimen and send to the lab. We can meet again next week and I will prescribe you a medication".

One week later.

Patient: "Hello Doctor, I am here again as we agreed."

Doctor: "Welcome, indeed I received the output from the lab. Your genetic data indicate as best options some compounds, and, paired with the clinical information

A. Serretti, MD, PhD (✉)
Department of Biomedical and Neuromotor Sciences, University of Bologna,
Viale Carlo Pepoli 5, Bologna 40123, Italy
e-mail: alessandro.serretti@unibo.it

J.K. Rybakowski, MD, PhD
Department of Adult Psychiatry, Poznan University of Medical Sciences,
ul.Szpitalna 27/33, Poznan 60-572, Poland
e-mail: janusz.rybakowski@gmail.com

© Springer International Publishing Switzerland 2016
J.K. Rybakowski, A. Serretti (eds.), *Genetic Influences on Response to Drug Treatment for Major Psychiatric Disorders*, DOI 10.1007/978-3-319-27040-1_7

I already collected, it seems that this is the most appropriate treatment for you. In fact it could lead to some unwanted side effects such as… and there is no guaranty of efficacy, but I would rate the expected global benefit above the other treatment options we have. See you next week and tell me how it is going."

There is no better way to clarify which are the clinical implications of pharmacogenetics than a narrative. Indeed what is reported above is not what could happen in the future, but what is already happening in many locations around the world. At present thousands of subjects have been treated according to pharmacogenetic indications, and, from what is reported in published papers, they received a relevant benefit in terms of efficacy and tolerability. The optimal drug is chosen at the beginning of the treatment, thus reducing the trial-and-error procedure routinely in use and reducing the time to improvement, with evident benefits for the individual suffering and the societal costs.

The aim of this final chapter is to discuss aspects related to what is described above, the clinical application of pharmacogenetics.

7.2 The Present Status of Pharmacogenetics in Practice

In the previous chapters, you were updated on the most recent scientific information in the field; as you may have noticed, there are good and bad news. Good news are the many DNA variants which have been found to be influencing efficacy and tolerability of many psychotropic drugs, at a variable degree of confidence. The bad news is exactly the same.

There are in fact too many variants affecting these traits; it is not therefore a straightforward prediction such as in other fields of medicine: "you have this variant and this drug is good/bad for you." Dozens of variants have shown to have a variable degree of influence on individual drug reactions but not a single one with a large and universal effect. Each one of the variants received at least one sample where the effect was not detectable, but on an aggregate level, each of them seems to have a little influence. Little influence means that a single variant does not dramatically change the individual reaction to treatment; thus they should be combined in a proper way in order to obtain a clinically useful tool, and the degree of confidence is also variable, with none achieving a high and unequivocal impact. Further genetic source of variants has not been much considered in literature. Apart from SNPs, there are many other sources of variation; without much detail, we should consider methylation, copy number variation, and de novo mutations, not to mention all possible modulating factors in the transcription process. Appropriate study design is also needed to progress our knowledge [2].

Therefore at present we are not sure which and how many of the variants listed in the previous chapters should be included in the practical screening tool; also we are not sure as well how they should be combined for a clear clinical indication. The most simple hypothesis is to make a summary, i.e., if a subject has 5HTTLPR long variant has an increased possibility to benefit from SSRIs, if the same subject has also the GNB3 rs5443 (C825T) T variant, the possibility to benefit from SSRIs is increased even more. But we are not sure yet that this is the correct strategy; possibly there is a ceiling effect and the combination of variants should not be linear but following a more specific model. At present this problem is faced by offering a warning or suggestion on groups of drugs based on the global genetic profile instead of offering indication for a specific compound..

In fact, there are only few cases in which the indication is clear and straightforward; first of all is the case of carbamazepine, unfortunately a drug not much used in psychiatry. In this case the FDA stated about 8 years ago in the drug label that: "Patients with ancestry in genetically at-risk populations [Asians] should be screened for the presence of hla-b*1502 prior to initiating treatment with tegretol. Patients testing positive for the allele should not be treated with tegretol unless the benefit clearly outweighs the risk" (http://www.accessdata.fda.gov/). This is a clear example how pharmacogenetics may help to reduce the risk of severe unwanted effects in the clinical practice. However apart from this very special case, the genetic indication for carbamazepine does not offer further help for efficacy or in other populations.

For other compounds the pharmacogenetic indication may, on the other hand, be useful for administering the appropriate dose, as you saw in the previous chapters. In fact genetic testing (CYP2D6 genotyping) is recommended also for pimozide (a first-generation antipsychotic) and some other ones. Indeed, in poor CYP2D6 metabolizers, pimozide doses should not exceed 0.05 mg/kg/day in children or 4 mg/day in adults, and doses should not be increased earlier than 14 days. Another indication to genotyping is provided for valproate prescription in children/adolescents (A467T and W748S polymorphisms in the POLG gene) to prevent the risk of liver toxicity FDA Label for valproic acid and OTC, POLG https://www.pharmgkb. org/label/PA166104825).

For all the other indications, as you saw in the various chapters, results at present are not that straightforward; also drug metabolizing enzymes, which are frequently mentioned by FDA in many drug labels, do not offer strong indications about how to adjust the dose for many compounds.

Nevertheless, an increasing amount of published papers report the benefit for using the pharmacogenetic strategy in the clinical practice all the same, even combining variants with algorithms that have a relatively low degree of confidence. In fact, as reported in some chapters, a number of tools are already available both at commercial level and at academic level. They vary largely in terms of composition and cost (we will discuss cost issues later on); moreover commercial tools do not reveal the algorithm used, since copyright protects it. This is an important limitation because replications can be performed only by the copyright owners and not by the whole scientific community. This has been suggested as a fact which should give much caution in interpreting the sometimes overly confident results reported by many companies. However we may not state that results are not valid; indeed a variable level of prediction has been repeatedly reported for many different products.

In our opinion the positive results reported are real; they are most probably due to what we can define as an average effect of the polymorphisms included in each tool. On the basis of decades of literature, it is now clear that not all variants modulate drug effects on all individuals, but this may be true for a part of subjects. Therefore, despite the fact that some genes do not exert any influence in the specific individual under exam, we may observe an aggregate effect on samples. Therefore the variant combination in each tool may change the rate of efficacy or tolerability at a population level, thus yielding a global benefit.

At this point, it is important to discuss which is the threshold for considering a benefit in clinical practice. An expensive tool which increases benefit or decreases possible unwanted side effects of few percent points may be not relevant; on the other hand, a striking effect has important individual, societal, and economic benefits.

Indeed, in the previous chapters, you saw that also a relatively small prediction benefit, in the range of 5–10 % toward a better outcome, may result in a relevant cost/benefit ratio. Most products claim effects larger than that.

As an example, GeneSight from Assurex, FDA approved, has been recently covered for payment by US Department of Veterans Affairs. The company claims that they manage about 300 samples per day.

It is a buccal swab identifying a combination of eight gene variants (CYP2D6, CYP2C19, CYP2C9, CYP3A4, CYP2B6, CYP1A2, 5-HTTLPR, and HTR2A) offering indications about (any) antidepressant efficacy and tolerability. The example is interesting because the GeneSight odds ratios are in the range 2–5, with a relevant economic benefit [4]. However similar broad effects have been reported also for other specific genes, such as ABCB1, but they are not commercially available at present. Another example is Genecept, which adds also genes for gated calcium channel, Ankyrin G, 5HT2C, DRD2, and MTHFR, other than 5-HTTLPR, CYP2D6, CYP2C19, and CYP3A4. This product informs also on the disease liability, not only drug response. In both cases, however, none of the included variants have been confirmed in all studies, but the company study claims a relevant population effect.

So, based on those figures, present pharmacogenetic products may be considered already useful, provided that the effects are replicated in a sufficient number of samples. Further, we may expect that with increasing knowledge of the involved variants and their combination, the benefit will increase steadily.

7.3 Problematic Practical Pharmacogenetic Issues

With the future spreading of pharmacogenetic tools in everyday clinical practice, a number of potentially problematic issues arise [1].

Let's start with the end point, the clinicians at the office as described at the beginning of the chapter. At present psychiatrists are not that familiar with medical devices, and also simple and basic routine laboratory tests are not performed in many cases. A large number of psychiatrists rely on the clinical interview which is followed by the drug prescription. This procedure has a great deal of variation, with much longer time spent with the patient in western countries compared to very short contacts in Asian countries. What is common is the general paucity of laboratory and medical exam requests; this is due to the little relevance so far for many psychiatric conditions.

The advent of pharmacogenetic tools requires therefore a change in the routine method of working. Psychiatrists should ask for a specific laboratory testing *before* prescription, and this also raises further problems discussed hereafter.

In practical terms, the clinician should ask for a specimen (saliva or blood), which should be sent to appropriate laboratories, or to send the subject to an equipped lab with the prescription. Then wait a few days for the response and see again the patient for the targeted prescription.

The procedure needed for clinical pharmacogenetics is therefore not without limitations; apart from direct costs, there is the issue of lag before the beginning of treatment. At present, samples must be shipped to equipped labs with the lab output received not sooner than a few days; in the case of very severe or suicidal subjects, this may be troublesome, also in terms of doctors' liability. Who is responsible for what may happen in the few days between the first and second contact? Obviously the doctor is; no informed consent may avoid this.

7.4   Cost, Benefit, and Stakeholders

Any new treatment or diagnostic test must undergo careful government evaluation before being paid to citizen in most countries. Pharmacogenetic tools therefore must demonstrate a relevant and sufficient benefit in order to be paid by stakeholders such as health national systems or insurances. In particular, in recent times, the economic crisis much tightened the authorization process in many countries.

At present, based on the considerations above, we are just on the threshold of this limit. As you saw in previous chapters, the prediction of single SNPs is not above few percent points in the response or side effect rate [3]. In fact, apart from the GeneSight test, which received some refund, there are no cases of approved and paid testing worldwide.

This scenario is likely to change in the future when cost/benefit analyses will evaluate next-generation tools with higher predictive capacities. The push in many research programs and funding agencies toward personalized treatment research is likely to move forward present knowledge leading to widespread clinical application.

Until then, however, the price of available tools is to be paid by the single subject or by research universities, thus much limiting the use.

This, despite the huge improvement that we could reach with a personalized prediction, is a relevant step after more than 50 years of psychotropic medication use.

Ideally, the combination of biomarkers other than DNA SNPs, as you saw in the specific chapter, could increase the clinical usefulness of the tool, but also in this case at increase of costs and time as we will discuss later.

7.5 An Integrated Prediction?

As you saw in the chapter about "Complementation of pharmacogenetics with biomarkers and neuroimaging," it is possible to use also complementary sources of information.

In fact, it is difficult to hypothesize that genes alone may offer a largely relevant clinical prediction. At best, according to various sources, the combined gene prediction may explain less than half of the variability to drug response. And this is only when all influencing variants are correctly identified and weighted in an appropriate model. Therefore it can be hypothesized that complementary sources of information may be used in the individual prediction before then. Possible complementary prediction tools include blood biomarkers and imaging. In this field of investigation, you have seen that the situation is similar to the one about SNP analysis: some results have been confirmed but none with sufficient evidence to guarantee a universal and stable prediction.

From a practical point of view, the blood biomarker analysis is a bit more complicated and costly compared to SNP analysis. The sample must be blood and not saliva; it needs a timely management in terms of storage at low temperatures, dedicated special and expensive tubes (at present about 15 euros each), and appropriate laboratories with expenses higher than SNP analysis particularly if the analysis is needed in real time for each subject. In fact, to our knowledge, the biomarker analysis has not been applied yet in clinical practice due to those limitations.

Imaging analysis poses even more complicated issues. As you can easily imagine, it is largely far from the clinical routine to administer a magnetic resonance in the 2–3 days after the psychiatric consultation. Apart from logistic issues and costs, there is also the problem of the interpretation of the drug prediction imaging results which is not at present common knowledge for general radiologists.

Further, the model including SNPs, blood biomarkers, and imaging results could be not manageable due to much complexity. How signals should be combined? It is already sufficiently complicated to combine SNPs; one can easily imagine the complexity of the three sets of data.

At present therefore the only integrated prediction we can suggest is the combination of SNP data with clinical data in order to obtain a comprehensive profile. If, as an example, a patient has a counterindication for drugs inducing weight gain, we will limit the choice among the ones with low weight gain effect. Then within those ones, we will select the one or two which are most indicated according to the SNP genetic analysis.

7.6 Concluding Remarks

Throughout the whole book, you have learned how far pharmacogenetics of psychotropic drugs has gone in a couple of decades of research. A relevant number of DNA SNP variants have been associated in many studies to drug response or tolerability. Personalized DNA prescription has also started to be used in clinical practice in a number of universities, and some companies are currently offering the service via web.

The benefit of pharmacogenetics is potentially huge in terms of subject reduced suffering and societal economic benefit. However the science behind it is still incomplete at best; clinicians are reluctant to use a tool they do not know well and stakeholders need strong science and data to allow for a widespread use.

We are at present therefore in a very exciting time where it is expected that in the next few years, the advancement in the knowledge of the specific DNA variant influence will lead to reliable, effective, and cheap tools for everyday routine use.

References

1. Howland RH (2014) Pharmacogenetic testing in psychiatry: not (quite) ready for primetime. J Psychosoc Nurs Ment Health Serv 52(11):13–16. doi:10.3928/02793695-20141021-09
2. Malhotra AK, Zhang JP, Lencz T (2012) Pharmacogenetics in psychiatry: translating research into clinical practice. Mol Psychiatry 17(8):760–769. doi:10.1038/mp.2011.146
3. Olgiati P, Bajo E, Bigelli M, De Ronchi D, Serretti A (2012) Should pharmacogenetics be incorporated in major depression treatment? Economic evaluation in high- and middle-income European countries. Prog Neuropsychopharmacol Biol Psychiatry 36(1):147–154
4. Winner JG, Carhart JM, Altar CA, Goldfarb S, Allen JD, Lavezzari G, Parsons KK, Marshak AG, Garavaglia S, Dechairo BM (2015) Combinatorial pharmacogenomic guidance for psychiatric medications reduces overall pharmacy costs in a 1 year prospective evaluation. Curr Med Res Opin 31(9):1633–1643. doi:10.1185/03007995.2015.1063483